THE
RESTAURANT COMPANION™
A guide to healthier eating out

Hope S. Warshaw, M.M.Sc., R.D.

SURREY BOOKS
101 East Erie Street
Suite 900
Chicago, Illinois 60611

THE RESTAURANT COMPANION[TM]**: A GUIDE TO HEALTHIER EATING OUT** is published by Surrey Books, Inc., 101 E. Erie Street, Suite 900, Chicago, IL 60611. "The Restaurant Companion" is a registered trade mark of Surrey Books, Inc.

This book is manufactured in the United States of America.

First edition. 1 2 3 4 5

Library of Congress Cataloging in Publication Data:
Warshaw, Hope S., 1954–
    The restaurant companion: a guide to healthier eating out / Hope S. Warshaw.
    p. 320 cm.
    ISBN 0-940625-13-X : $9.95
    1. Nutrition–Handbooks, manuals, etc.
2. Restaurants, lunch rooms, etc.–United States–Handbooks, manuals, etc.   1. Title.
RA784.W365   1990   89-21733
613.2–dc20   CIP

Single copies may be ordered directly from the publisher. Send $11.95 (check or money order) per book, which includes postage and handling, to Surrey Books at the address above. The Surrey Books Catalog is also available, free of charge, from the publisher.

Editorial Production: Bookcrafters, Inc., Chicago.
Art Direction and Design: Hughes & Co., Chicago.
Illustrations: Elizabeth Allen.

CONTENTS

Foreword by Dr. George L. Blackburn V

1 Healthier Eating Out: A Practice Whose Time Has Come 1

2 Skills and Strategies for Restaurant Eating 6

3 How to Eat Out with *The Restaurant Companion* 21

4 Mexican Style 29

5 Chinese Style 47

6 Seafood Style 67

7 Italian Style 85

8 Thai Style 107

9 Japanese Style 127

10 Indian Style 146

11 Middle Eastern Style 166

12 French/Continental Style 185

13 American Style 206

14 Fast Food Style 226

15 Salad Bar Style 249

16 Luncheon Style 261

17 Breakfast and Brunch 282

18 Airline Style 300

19 Choosing Beverages: Alcoholic and Non-Alcoholic 306

To . . .
my wonderful (and ever-expanding) family,
fabulously supportive friends, and
clients from whom I've learned more
than textbooks could ever teach

Acknowledgments . . .

A big thanks to those people at Surrey Books: Publisher Susan Schwartz, who recognized the need for this book and her continued enthusiasm about its publication; Margaret Liddiard, whose marketing skills are appreciated and whose sense of humor kept me laughing; Gene DeRoin, my editor, whose patience and perseverance to complete this book were unending; and Sally Hughes, who so ably designed the covers and interior.

Another big thanks to the people at *Diabetes Self-Management,* R.A. Rappaport Publishing, Inc. To Robert Dinsmoor, under whose editorial direction the "Eating Out" column was initiated, and to Rena Springer and James Hazlett who provided continued editorial assistance to the column, which has appeared for two years in this bi-monthly magazine.

My thanks also to Dr. George L. Blackburn for willingly writing the "Foreword" to *The Restaurant Companion.*

Foreword

Dining out, ordering out, and, indeed, eating any food prepared by others—apart from our own control—poses a major challenge to healthy eating. Given the difficulty of recognizing low-fat, high-fiber foods, it is no wonder that restaurant eating is commonly the downfall of many people trying to improve their health by eating right.

With *The Restaurant Companion,* the challenge of eating out can be transformed into an opportunity to learn about selecting optimal foods, to relax when eating out, and to enjoy life more through healthier dining habits.

Hope Warshaw has all the credentials for preparing this nutritional guide. She has devoted years to working with both individuals and groups to change their diet through healthy food selection and, thereby, avoid diet-related medical conditions such as diabetes, cardiovascular disease, hypertension, and obesity. She has focused this book on a major requisite for successful eating: how to choose wisely when dining in restaurants.

People need to vary their diets and enjoy eating without developing a tolerance—and craving—for foods that lead to an increased consumption of fat, sugar, and salt while reducing their interest in fruits and vegetables. Ironically, most people eat less than 20 types of food during any one season of the year. The end result is, of course, overeating and overweight, as well as missed opportunities to use diet to improve health and the enjoyment of life.

New restaurant experiences, new foods, and new eating patterns can break up this routine. Proper meal choices in restaurants can be healthy and enjoyable while providing a break from busy lifestyles. The unlimited opportunities for healthier eating made possible by the diverse restaurants around the country are brought out in *The Restaurant Companion*.

Indeed, this book is a great starting place for you and your friends to experience just how good—and how healthy—restaurant food can be when ordered by an informed consumer. It also provides an excellent opportunity to become acquainted with a host of European and Asian cuisines that offer a wide variety of foods to replace our traditional eating patterns— standard meals that offer no new tastes or textures and usually employ foods with far too much sugar, oil, and protein. The new and unique approaches to healthier eating in *The Restaurant Companion* can also be used at the much-frequented fast food spots, salad bars, sandwich shops—even when flying!

Soon, you will be adopting the healthy changes discovered in this book for your own diet and advocating them to family and friends. And with the confidence you gain by accepting the restaurant challenge, you may find yourself dining out more frequently and enjoying a wide variety of foods more.

George L. Blackburn, M.D., Ph.D.
Chief, Nutrition/Metabolism Laboratory,
New England Deaconess Hospital
Associate Professor of Surgery,
Harvard Medical School

1

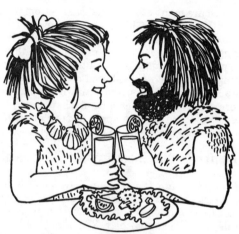

Healthier Eating Out

A practice whose time has come

T his book is intended to become one of your dining companions. It can accompany you to the restaurant or be consulted prior to leaving home. It can be used to determine which foods you'd be best off ordering and which to avoid in an Italian, Chinese, Mexican, and many other kinds of restaurants. It will prove helpful whether you simply want to eat healthier or are closely modifying one or several aspects of your diet.

It also will give you an idea of the types of foods you will find in a Thai, Japanese, or Middle Eastern dining spot (among others) and which of these are your best bets for health.

The Restaurant Companion provides realistic advice and practical guidelines for eating in the wide variety of restaurants found in America today. It covers eating places from inexpensive to costly, from casual to elegant, and from the usual to the more esoteric. Included are many ethnic restaurants—from the ubiquitous Italian and Chinese places to the less frequented Indian and Thai establishments. Beyond giving guidelines for ethnic dining spots, this book also provides information for authentically American eating places such as fast food chains, family style restaurants, salad bars, and eating on airplanes. The information in each restaurant chapter is easy to understand and easy to apply to both everyday experiences and those once-in-a-while special occasions.

Who needs **The Restaurant Companion?**

The Restaurant Companion: A Guide to Healthier Eating Out was written for a wide array of people. The book can be valuable to anyone who simply has made the decision to eat healthier. You might not have any medical problems for which you have been told to restrict certain foods but nevertheless have made a commitment to yourself to do all that you can to adopt a healthy lifestyle. As part of the plan, you are trying to minimize fat, cholesterol, and sodium intake. Your changes in eating habits are likely to be balanced with exercise to keep you in shape and burn off some excess calories.

This book is also written for people who must restrict their dietary intake due to specific medical problems. There has been much attention in the last several years to the relationship between elevated blood cholesterol and the increased risk of heart attack. For this reason, people are now encouraged to limit fats, saturated fat, and dietary cholesterol. This book provides you with lots of information on how to continue to enjoy dining out while following a meal plan that leads to that goal!

The Restaurant Companion can also be helpful to those among us who are trying to lose weight, as it encourages a low-fat, calorie-conscious approach to eating out. Many people tend to avoid eating out while "on a diet." But if you are like many Americans and eating out is part of your usual game plan, you are likely to resume the practice "after the diet." So why not take this opportunity to learn how you can continue to enjoy restaurant dining and lose weight at the same time. After all, the same basic principles that apply to weight loss, low fat intake, and portion control apply to long-term weight maintenance.

The Restaurant Companion is also ideal for people who actually have achieved long-sought weight loss. It will provide ways for them to enjoy some of the foods they may have missed while teaching them which foods to continue to limit and which to eat very sparingly. It will introduce dieters and those interested in weight maintenance to many new behaviors and strategies that combine the fun of dining out with the wisdom of calorie-conscious eating.

This guide will also assist people with diabetes, whether they are on insulin or not. Today, people with both insulin-dependent and non-insulin-dependent diabetes are being encouraged to follow meal plans that are quite similar to the way all Americans are being urged to eat. Generally speaking, this amounts to a moderate carbohydrate, high fiber, low fat, and relatively low protein intake. Many people with adult onset diabetes are overweight, and therefore the recommendations provided here for monitoring calorie and fat consumption are quite appropriate. Specific attention is given to those with concerns about diabetes by providing sample meals in the restaurant chapters that are in accordance with diabetes meal planning recommendations from the American Diabetes Association.

This book can also be used by those who have been encouraged to limit sodium intake due to high blood pressure or other medical conditions. Specific information is provided on ways to keep sodium content at a minimum in certain types of restaurants. Ordering models are provided throughout the book for those trying to limit their sodium consumption.

So, if you want to continue dining out *and* enjoying it but realize that there are many not-so-nutritious food choices out there, this book will be a useful guide. Whether you simply want to learn about healthier eating out or are managing a medical condition by modifying your diet, *The Restaurant Companion* can help.

Learning how to eat out healthier

The premise that eating out must always lead to overeating or a dietary disaster has no basis in fact. *The Restaurant Companion* will show you how easy healthier eating out can be. All you need do is follow a few simple guidelines and begin practicing some tricks of the trade, all of which will be discussed in the next chapter. Of course, one of the most important aspects of learning how to eat out healthier is self-responsibility. In other words, *you* have control over whether or not you choose to eat healthier and stay on track with your nutritional goals. Rest assured, it is quite possible, even easy, once you have your priorities set.

For starters, you must be willing and wanting. Willing to give up some of the high fat, great-tasting nutritional disasters and trade them in for just as tasty, healthier foods. Compare, for instance, a Mexican chimichanga—a deep-fried flour tortilla filled with spicy ground beef and cheese—with a soft taco filled with the same spicy beef and cheese. The same filling is used in both, but the soft taco is not deep fried and therefore a healthier food choice, although you enjoy the same hot Mexican spiciness. Eating healthier does not mean eating bland, untasty foods. It's simply a matter of combining "tasty" with "healthy."

Wanting is the other half. You must have the desire or motivation to choose healthier foods. Maybe you simply want to feel that you are feeding youself in a healthier way. Maybe you have assessed your present habits and realize that your fat intake is excessive. You might be motivated due to medical reasons. Perhaps you've discovered that your blood cholesterol is elevated or that you have high blood pressure and have been encouraged to reduce your sodium intake. For whatever reasons, eating healthier is a positive change for today and in the long run.

There are certainly many people today who follow particular meal plans or special diets either out of choice or due to medical necessity. Unfortunately, it is all too common that people who are educated about following special diets receive very little, if any, information on maintaining their meal plan in restaurants. Even more unfortunate is the fact that people in general are not even provided with sufficient information to properly prepare a special diet at home. This is often due to very little or no time spent with a registered dietitian, learning how to modify their present habits to manage one or a variety of medical problems.

The reality is that many people eat out often. Yet few have developed strategies for making sure restaurant meals contribute to their health and well-being. Too often, if any guidelines for restaurant eating are available, they are quite rigid, often just for American fare, and relatively unrealistic. For example, a suggestion often heard is to use tomato juice or consommé as an appetizer. Now with all of the great-tasting foods listed on a menu, who is going to be satisfied with these bland, unadventurous suggestions? What often happens when you are provided with such information is that you stick with the rigid guidelines for a while, then get very tired of the regimentation. You decide that you want Chinese food and proceed to abandon better judgment and order whatever strikes your fancy.

When provided with solid information on what to order and what to avoid you can make sensible—and interesting—choices from virtually any menu. Furthermore, you will feel more comfortable making these decisions and be more willing to adhere to your nutrition plan. It is vitally important to believe that you have some options. If not, it becomes quite difficult to stay on track when out-of-the-ordinary situations occur.

If you are going to eat out, and there is no reason why you should not, you need practical information and realistic guidelines. You need to know which dishes are wise choices when you go into an Italian or Chinese restaurant; you might want to know how to approach a salad bar or how to order in a fast food chain. Or maybe you wonder if being on a low cholesterol and low saturated fat diet will permit you to eat Thai or Indian food. Basically, it is our philosophy that whether you are simply watching calories or are learning to control your diabetes, it is in your power to make the kind of wise food choices that will allow you to eat in almost any restaurant. Go ahead, be adventurous. Experiment with the knowledge gained from this book.

2

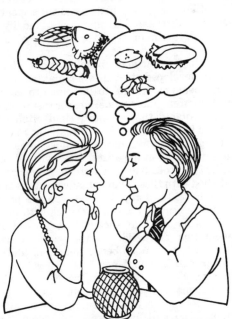

Skills and Strategies
For restaurant eating

Whether you're lavishing for three hours over a very expensive meal in a French cafe or simply rushing through one of the many fast food franchises for a 15-minute lunch on the run, the principles of healthy eating out remain the same. In fact, the basic tenets for healthy restaurant eating, albeit with a few extra precautions and recommendations, are generally the same as those for healthful eating at home.

SIX SKILLS

The six basic skills needed for healthier dining out are not complicated: 1) monitor the frequency of eating out; 2) choose the restaurant carefully; 3) make wise menu selections; 4) monitor the fats; 5) make special requests; and 6) practice portion control. These watchwords will be revisited time and time again in the chapters of this book. If practiced, they will assist you in any eating situation. So read on carefully, then apply the six watchwords, whether you're eating sushi, enchiladas, moo shi chicken, pizza, or a good old American hamburger.

1. Monitor the frequency of eating out

Even though it is quite possible to eat healthy and, if necessary, stay on course with a special meal plan at any eating establishment, it is often more difficult than when eating at home. You certainly don't have as much control over what goes into the food as you do in your own kitchen. Beyond not having as much control, restaurants offer taste treats that whet your appetite. Treats are more difficult to avoid when you can simply open your mouth and request that these items arrive at your table. For these reasons, it is important to monitor the frequency with which you eat out.

The more frequently you eat out, the more you need to closely monitor your choices and portions. Many people find themselves eating lunch out five days a week and then dinner out one or two times a week. If you cast all caution to the wind on all of these occasions, you will likely suffer health consequences in years to come, not to mention packing on pounds in the near future. However, if you are at home during the week for lunch or take a brown bag to work and you dine out biweekly, you probably can take a bit more liberty in your food choices.

Another factor in monitoring the frequency of eating out is consideration of your specific nutrition goals. If you are simply attempting to eat healthier by cutting down on fats, cholesterol, and salt and you don't eat out that frequently, you can allow yourself a bit more liberty in restaurants. However, if you must monitor your saturated fat, cholesterol, and sodium intake due to known heart disease or high blood cholesterol, it will be important to control more strictly your food choices, extra fats, and portion sizes. So be clear about your health and nutrition goals and establish a frequency of eating out that fits your lifestyle and health goals.

2. *Choose the restaurant carefully*

The first order of business prior to dining out is to choose an establishment that serves foods you can eat. Be careful that you don't find yourself in a place with a very limited menu from which there are simply no choices. A fried chicken or fish and chips fast-food stop would be a good example. There are simply no good selections at those places. Choosing an appropriate restaurant might require some assertiveness if you are with a group of people. It is important that you let your needs be known in a clear and positive way.

In most instances you will be familiar with the menu because you have eaten there previously or in another location of that particular chain. Or maybe you've been told about the restaurant by friends or have heard about it through advertising. In the rare instance when you are completely unfamiliar with what to expect, you have the option of calling to ask some questions. Try to determine if there are some menu selections consistent with your health goals. Ask if you can request special preparation. Is the chef willing to leave off a sauce or gravy? Can the chef steam or broil fish rather than fry it? Will they omit some high-sodium seasonings if requested? Don't forget, you are anonymous when you call, so ask what you want. Today, there are many more people concerned about what they eat, and most restaurants are pleased to grant reasonable requests. They want pleased customers and they want you back at their tables again and again.

3. *Make wise menu selections*

The biggest challenge to the health-conscious diner is to peruse the menu selections and come up with an order that is both satisfying to the taste buds and at the same time meets your nutritional needs. Most menus will represent a cross-section of good choices and poor choices. The challenge of making appropriate decisions can be especially difficult when you are very hungry and your resistance to "danger" foods is low.

A word of caution: do not set yourself up for over-eating and/or eating the wrong foods by starving during the day to "save calories" for the restaurant later. In addition to simply responding to hunger pangs, it is easier to rationalize extras if you think you have previously eaten such a small amount that a little more of this or that high-fat and high-calorie food will not make a difference. Unfortunately, this balance never seems to equalize in the end. More times than not, you will eat foods you should avoid and more of them than you need.

When making menu choices, it's best to decide first on the main focus, usually the entree. It might occur that a particular starch or vegetable is served with an entree, and that will affect your decision about what you order in addition. For instance, a casserole dish might contain vegetables, whereas another selection might be served only with rice pilaf and you can make the additional choice of a salad or vegetable. Or maybe you've decided to splurge a bit on the entree, and that will influence your decision whether or not to have an appetizer or soup. In many eating situations, such as a fast-food meal, a simple lunch, or pizza and salad, the focus is clearer. There are fewer decisions to make because there are really no extras.

Each of the restaurant chapters is set up to assist you in making wise menu selections. You will first be provided with some general nutrition guidelines about that particular cuisine; then you will look over a typical menu, including both healthful and not-so-healthful choices; finally, you will see model meals, derived from the menu, that will help you order to achieve particular nutrition goals such as controlling calories, fat, cholesterol, or sodium.

4. Monitor the fats

Whether you are simply trying to eat healthier, trying to lower your cholesterol, or managing your diabetes, one of the goals in wise menu selection is to consume less fat. Choosing menu items to minimize fat intake in a restaurant setting is a skill to develop. Fat is used to enhance taste and flavor. It certainly does that, whether it be butter, margarine, cream, or bacon. However, while enhancing flavor, fat adds significant calories, often without adding any food volume. Consider the medium baked potato, which contains about 100 calories. Add to that 1 teaspoon of stick margarine and 2 tablespoons of sour cream, and you have another 100 calories with no increased food volume. Fats, depending on which type, may also contribute saturated fat and cholesterol – unwanted additions to your diet.

Fat creeps into restaurant selections in a variety of ways. For starters, at more upscale establishments bread and butter or crackers and cheese spread often greet you at the table. Appetizers are frequently fried or contain high-fat ingredients (think about fried mozzarella sticks on an Italian menu or fried jumbo shrimp in a Chinese restaurant). Entree choices, such as duck or prime rib, may be high in fat before any ingredients are even added during food preparation. Fat is often added in the form of butter, cream, sour cream, cheese, mayonnaise, and cooking oil. Entrees may be fried or sauteed, thus incorporating varying quantities of fat in the cooking process. Once the food arrives at the table, the American way is to add yet more fat in the form of salad dressing to salads, butter to vegetables, sour cream to potatoes, or melted cheese dip to nachos. Dessert is another course where lots of fat is found – consider ice cream, chocolate mousse, or cheesecake.

Granted, many foods contain fat, and many preparation methods add lots of fat, saturated fat, and cholesterol. But there are also many selections that represent healthier choices. Successful restaurant diners are able to pick and choose among the array of items to find tasty and healthy foods to eat. Consider the following example, with menu items taken from a mid-priced American hamburger and sandwich restaurant:

High Fat/Calorie Choices	**Lower Fat/Calorie Choices**
Potato skins filled with melted Cheddar cheese and topped with bacon bits (2 skins)	Cup of chicken-vegetable soup Small salad with Italian dressing served on the side (1 tbsp.)

Cheeseburger smothered with sauteed onions and peppers French fries	Ham sandwich served on rye bread with mustard
Total calories: 900	580
% of calories as fat: 56	40
Goal for % of calories as fat 30	30

This example demonstrates that different foods chosen from the same menu can differ significantly in fat and calorie content. Throughout this book, comparisons will be made between healthier and not-so-healthy choices. You'll be able to see how just a few simple changes here and there can make substantial differences in fat, cholesterol, and sodium consumption.

Fat is the most saturated form of calories consumed. Volume being equal, carbohydrate and protein foods have about half the calories of fat. For this reason, it is extremely important that you become a good fat detector, finding ways to pay careful attention to all the ways in which fat creeps into restaurant foods.

Beyond simply knowing which foods are high in fat, there are descriptive words used to describe the preparation of menu items. Some of these words should become "Red Flags," signals to you that this selection is not a good choice due to excessive fat. Examples of Red Flag words are "fried," "deep fried," "breaded and fried," "stuffed," and so on. Each ethnic cuisine and style of cooking incorporates fats in different ways. The restaurant chapters will note the Red Flag words to monitor for that particular type of cuisine. On the positive side, there are many "Green Flags" to look for, which indicate low-fat foods or low-fat food preparation methods. Green Flag words include "steamed," "poached," "blackened," "mesquite-grilled," "stir-fried," and others. The Green Flag words will also be noted in each restaurant chapter.

5. Make special requests

Sometimes it is necessary to make special requests in order to have what you want and need. If your special requests are reasonable and asked for in a friendly yet assertive manner, you will most likely have them granted. Obviously, in some situations, such as at a fast-food chain at lunch time, it is more difficult to make special requests. But in most dining situations special requests are quite appropriate.

There are several thoughts and hints to keep in mind to bolster your confidence. First, you are paying for the meal, and you have the privilege, if you are being reasonable, to have food prepared the way you desire. You may request that the chef leave something off or reduce the quantity of a particular item. In essence, it is costing the restaurant less to serve you. Second, most businesses want and need your patronage. It is probable that if your special requests are courteously granted and you are pleased with the results, you will return and—better yet—refer friends and family. Third, waitpersons are used to special requests today because more people are carefully watching the foods they consume both at and away from home. I'm in restaurants a lot and hear more and more people ask about the particulars of what's in a dish and if this or that can be changed.

Special requests may encompass asking for a substitution. For example, you would rather have a baked potato than French fries, or you would rather have mustard on a sandwich than the "special sauce," which is mayonnaise-based. A special request may be serving something on the side, such as salad dressing, a sauce, or gravy. Putting a high-fat or high-sodium item on the side allows you, the consumer, to control how much is used rather than the chef or waitperson. You might request that an item be broiled dry rather than drenched in butter or that a Chinese dish cooked in a wok be prepared with less oil or soy sauce.

Special requests also involve asking that something be left out of a dish because it will raise the sodium or fat level. For instance, sour cream or guacamole are added to many Mexican items; they can easily be left off. You might request that high-sodium items such as pickles or a high-fat and high-sodium item such as potato chips be eliminated from the plate. It is best that these items are not presented to you. They will be easier to avoid that way and you won't have to stare at them on your plate. Another special request, if your dining partners are willing, is to have items removed from the table. Usually, these are foods that greet you at your table without ordering: bread and butter, crackers and cheese spread, or tortilla chips and salsa at a Mexican restaurant. These potentially high-fat and high-sodium delights are easier to avoid if they are out of sight and out of mind.

As you make special requests more frequently, you will become more comfortable with the idea that you are not ruffling any feathers. When you initiate this practice, think of using phrases such as: "Do you think the chef would be able to . . . ," "I'd really appreciate it if you would . . . ," "Can I get . . . on the side?" If you need more ammunition, you may need to rely on medical reasons: "I am on a special meal plan," "I am under a doctor's care to restrict . . . ." The line that seems to be most effective in producing the desired results is: "I have an allergy to . . . ." No one wants you to have an allergic reaction right in their restaurant! Most restaurant chapters have a list of special requests that might assist you in ordering that particular cuisine.

6. *Practice portion control*

Once you have placed your order, the next step in healthy restaurant eating is to control the amount of food that is consumed. Unfortunately, you are served more food than you need more times than not. Picture yourself in a dining situation where you have just had your properly ordered meal served. Consider, for example, a poached salmon entree. In many restaurants the dinner portion would be at least 6–8 ounces cooked. This could be double what you should be eating. You know you should not become a member of the Clean Plate Club, yet it is easy to rationalize eating more of a food you know is good for you.

It is difficult to practice portion control but not impossible, and practice makes perfect. There are several strategies for managing these situations. "Doggie bags" have become more acceptable as people become more conscious of limiting excess quantities. Most restaurants have "doggie bags" available and are more than happy to give you one or to wrap extras up in aluminum foil.

One effective portion-control strategy is to ask for a "doggie bag" when your meal is *served* and to immediately portion out what you will eat in the restaurant and what you will take home. The theory "out of sight, out of mind" is quite helpful in practicing portion control. Sometimes "doggie bags" are unavailable or the situation does not lend itself to this request, for instance, at a business luncheon. If that is the case, try simply to portion out what you should eat, and separate that from the rest of the food. Place the portion not to be eaten on the side of your plate or on a bread or salad plate. If you are comfortable doing it, graciously offer a taste to your dining companions. Or put the portion you don't want to eat in the middle of the table, out of harm's way.

Sharing menu selections is another strategy to implement portion control. This requires one or more willing dining partners. You might want to try sharing an appetizer, salad, and entree and then have enough room to split a dessert. In some steak restaurants it's appropriate to have one person order the meal, which includes a steak, a large baked potato, and a trip to the salad bar. The other person can simply order a trip to the salad bar, and you both split the steak and baked potato. In some types of restaurants it is routine for people to share entrees; we have all followed such protocol when eating Chinese, Thai, Japanese, or pizza. In sharing situations be sure to make your food desires known to your eating partners to see if they are agreeable.

When initially practicing the above skills, it is difficult to forget the messages you heard during childhood about becoming a member of the Clean Plate Club or about the starving children in India, Africa, or whatever country your parents chose to select. Granted, no one is encouraging the waste of food, but it is important to ask yourself whether it is better for your health if the food is eaten or left on the plate. In either event, it won't reach any starving children. If weight control is your priority, you might wish to keep the following question in mind: is it better for the food to go to waste or to your waist?

FIVE STRATEGIES

In many cases, it is necessary to revise current behaviors and attitudes about eating in general and dining out in particular if one's culinary experiences are to change for the healthier. There are many strategies and tactics to help you do this, and the following five are among the most important: 1) develop a healthy mindset; 2) utilize preplanning; 3) modify eating behavior; 4) redefine fullness; and 5) enjoy the non-food pleasantries. Over time, these strategies will become routine and eating healthier will become much easier.

It is important for you to be clear with yourself and others around you that your intention is to change some eating habits. If you say one thing and do another, it is more difficult for people to support you in your efforts. Don't forget, actions speak louder than words.

1. Develop a healthy mindset

There are certain dangerous mindsets or preconceived notions about dining out that can easily lead to poor choices and overeating. It's important to determine what yours are, slowly extinguish these existing notions, and move on to a healthier mindset. One common dangerous mindset about dining out is that eating out is a special occasion, even though you do it two or three times per week. "Special occasion" to some means they can choose whatever their taste buds desire and eat until they're stuffed.

Another detrimental behavior is to watch yourself at home and then cast all caution to the wind and "pig out" in the restaurant. Treating yourself "well" becomes synonymous with having what you want even though it might be harmful to your health. Food is often used as a reward—you've had a rough day, which translates into deserving fried appetizers or a decadent chocolate dessert. Food is also used to celebrate—it's a child's birthday, a friend received a promotion—and again these situations are translated into "pigging out," which is rationalized for that particular occasion. Unfortunately, the occasions often become frequent events.

Another set of notions about eating out concerns getting your money's worth. The attitude of "I'm paying for it so I might as well eat it" is a dangerous mindset that again only leads to overeating. This attitude is one reason to avoid "all you can eat" places and "price fixed" menus where everything is included from soup to nuts. One thinks that not eating a part of the meal means not getting one's money's worth. This mindset is also easy to fall prey to when you are requesting that some item be left off the order or when food is left on the table or on your plate. The Clean Plate Club is not a club in which you want to continue your membership.

To be a successful restaurant diner, it is important to be honest about your present mindset for dining out. Determine if your attitudes work for you or against you. Work on changing those that you feel are detrimental to your goal of healthy eating.

After you have honestly assessed your present attitudes, you are ready to move on and establish new ones. First, it is important to be clear that eating healthy and/or paying attention to medical conditions are priorities. It is more important to keep your weight, cholesterol, and blood pressure under control than to eat what, how, and when you want. Second, it is most important that you believe you can continue to enjoy dining out while enjoying healthier foods. Enjoyment is key; people do not continue to practice behaviors that are not positively reinforced. Unpleasantness is avoided whenever there's a choice.

It is important to be clear with dining partners about your intention to eat healthy. Your decision might affect the choice of restaurant or the choice of menu items selected if you are ordering as a group. It will certainly be helpful to gain the support of people around you, but don't expect to get it all the time. There will be some, maybe your old eating buddies, who will not be pleased with your new attitudes and behaviors. Be on the ready for their statements goading you to deviate from your plan.

Lastly, think about changing the value of the meal from a dollars-and-cents perspective to whether you enjoyed what you ordered, feel satiated, and took pleasure in the total eating experience. Think about accentuating the environment.

2. Utilize preplanning

There is a preplanning concept taught in weight control called "calorie banking." Calorie banking teaches people to think about their food intake more than one meal at a time or, if necessary, more than one day at a time. For example, if you know that you will be celebrating an occasion at a fancy restaurant, think about "banking," or saving, some calories for that meal through the day, or even starting the day before. Over the course of a week, some occasions may be planned for higher calorie consumption, perhaps on weekends (when people tend to do more eating out), social events, or just to satisfy general food desires. Conversely, some times can be low-calorie days.

Another strategy for keeping your calorie account balanced is to add more exercise to your daily routine. Increasing the calories used means you put more calories back in the bank. If the bank account is "balanced" at the end of the week, your weight should stay even. If you're overdrawn, you know the results. Sorry, there's no overdraft protection at this bank.

This same concept can be applied if you are watching cholesterol, sodium, saturated fat, or other dietary components. For instance, if you know you're going out for high-sodium Chinese or Japanese food, make an effort to choose low-sodium foods during the day. Then at the restaurant you have a bit more leeway, yet your sodium bank will remain balanced.

One trap you might fall into, which often backfires, is eating so little prior to going out that you are starving, ready to eat anything that doesn't move once you are seated. This behavior is clearly a set-up to overeat. For one thing, you are extremely hungry so your resistance to off-limits foods is weakened. The other factor is that rationalizing extras is easier. You figure you've eaten so little that a bit more of this or that food won't do any harm. Unfortunately, more times than not, starving prior to eating out backfires. You are better off using the sensible banking approach, which calls for moderately decreasing the consumption beforehand of whichever dietary component(s) you are monitoring.

Another preplanning concept that may prove helpful is to have a good idea of what you will order prior to arriving at the restaurant. For the most part, you will be visiting eating establishments you already have been to or, if not, you have a good sense of what will be offered. For example, when you open most Chinese restaurant menus you will find similar listings of hot-and-sour soup, steamed white rice, chicken and broccoli, shrimp with assorted vegetables, and many other dishes whether you are in Boston, Chicago, or San Francisco. If you plan your order in advance, you are less tempted by smells, wandering eyes, and the menu listings.

Another strategy you can use in a restaurant that you visit frequently is simply not to look at the menu. This avoids a lot of taste bud fantasies and self-torture with "should I" or "shouldn't I" questions. Have your mind made up prior to arriving, and just don't open the menu when it is presented. Another helpful tactic is to try to order first so you don't talk yourself out of your plan or rationalize extras after you hear your dining partners place their orders.

When you are deciding on your menu choices, if soups and/or salads are available, think about using these as fillers. This is helpful if you have arrived very hungry. A cup of brothy soup or a nice crunchy green salad might just take the edge off your appetite. This strategy may help you fill up on healthier foods and be more successful in limiting portions later in the meal. This tactic is especially useful if your dining companions are ordering high-fat appetizers. Consider enjoying a spicy cup of very low-calorie and low-fat gazpacho (cold tomato soup) while the others are filling up on high-fat and high-cholesterol fried mozzarella sticks.

3. Modify eating behavior

Once you are served, several strategies may be practiced. Try to eat slowly and enjoy the foods you have selected. For the most part, people eat too fast and barely give their taste buds a chance to notice what is passing by. Keep in mind that it takes approximately 20 minutes for your stomach to notify your brain that you are full. So if you typically eat fast and finish a meal in 10 minutes, you've got 10 more minutes left before signals of fullness reach your brain. A lot of overeating can go on in those 10 minutes. If possible, try to keep pace with a dining partner who is eating slowly. Try to be the last one to finish.

Slowing the pace of eating is assisted by putting down your utensils frequently. Take a few bites, place the knife and fork by the side of your plate, and enjoy the taste sensations. Another way to slow eating is to stop for frequent sips of your beverage. This achieves two goals: it helps slow the pace of eating, and the additional fluids fill you up.

In many restaurants you will be served more food than you need. It is very difficult to make the decision not to eat any more when the food is sitting in front of you. You are pleasantly full, but you know there's room for more. It's time to practice the strategies of portion control that were discussed earlier. In addition to those tactics, also try to get into the habit of leaving a few bites on your plate. This helps to break the behavior of associating fullness and the end of a meal with a sparkling clean plate. It also may help you focus on your body's signals of fullness rather than letting the clean plate make the determination. Another strategy to put into practice is to signal the waitperson to remove your plate from the table. That will assist you in not overeating simply because the food is still in front of you.

4. Redefine fullness

Being clear about your definition of fullness is vital. Unfortunately, most people respond to external rather than internal cues. If you define fullness as that post-Thanksgiving-dinner bloated feeling, you are likely overeating quite frequently. If you use a clean plate and/or no food left on the table as your frame of reference for fullness, you're likely overeating as well. If you observe that your reference point for fullness is leading you to overeat, it's obviously time to establish a new definition.

The first challenge is to learn to listen to your internal signals. How does your stomach feel when you have had enough to eat? Begin to understand this sensation as a message to put down your knife and fork rather than wait for the old stuffed feeling. The second challenge is to slow the pace of eating. This allows your body more time to recognize fullness. Third, take time to think about and enjoy what you are eating. These strategies can help increase your feeling of satiety, which makes limiting portions easier.

5. Enjoy the non-food pleasantries

Frequently, you find yourself so focused on the food due to time constraints, hunger, or other stresses that enjoying the environment around you is missed. If you train yourself to enjoy all aspects of the eating experience, it will be easier to limit portions. Obviously, this strategy is not workable when you are cruising by the drive-in window of a fast-food chain to pick up your lunch, which you will guzzle down in 10 minutes on your way to your next appointment. Nevertheless, it's extremely important to provide yourself a few minutes of relaxation at mealtimes, even if you are in a hurry and the main purpose of eating is to refuel.

When you are dining out, try to enjoy the non-food niceties of the situation. Let yourself enjoy a few

Skills and Strategies

minutes of relaxation, concentrate on the conversation you're involved in, look around and enjoy the environment, observe the people in your midst. Enjoy being waited on. Think about not having to cook, put away leftovers, clear the table, or wash the dishes. Simply put, try to look beyond the food.

3

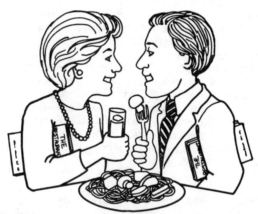

How to Eat Out
with
The Restaurant Companion

T
he *Restaurant Companion: A Guide to Healthier Eating Out* is designed to provide a very simple "hands-on" approach to feeling comfortable and relaxed while making wise and healthy food choices in any type of restaurant. A large portion of this book is devoted to providing you with practical and specific information about dining out.

The many restaurant chapters go into detail about particular categories of foods and cover America's most frequented types of eating places, including Chinese, Italian, fast food, Mexican, American family style, seafood, salad bars, brunch spots, airplane fare, and others. Less familiar ethnic restaurants are not overlooked: Thai, Japanese, Indian, Middle Eastern, and more are included.

In the restaurant section of the book each chapter is introduced with an overview of information about that type of cuisine. You'll find details on both the usual and unusual ingredients used, techniques of cooking, and the particular serving styles unique to that cuisine. Many of the chapters on eating in ethnic restaurants also contain interesting tidbits of information, such as the history of the cuisine, how it has evolved over time, significant details about preparation, and how a particular ethnic cooking style may have become Americanized.

Along with specific information about each cuisine and type of eating establishment, *The Restaurant Companion* provides you with lots of very practical suggestions for making wise selections from the menu. For this reason, you should literally make the book one of your restaurant companions. You may wish to keep it by your side in the restaurant and consult it as needed.

What to consider before ordering

An important section of each chapter provides you with information about the nutritional pros and cons of each restaurant's repertory. Guidelines are given to assist you in navigating your way around the menu when eating that particular fare. Strategies to keep your fat and cholesterol intake limited, to keep sodium down, and to minimize portions are provided in each chapter. When using this information, keep your personal dietary goals in mind. For instance, if you need to limit dietary cholesterol due to an elevated blood cholesterol level, pay special attention to comments about which foods are better or worse choices with reference to cholesterol content.

You also will find specific comments alerting you to which food items should be ordered or avoided if you are attempting to modify one or several dietary components—cholesterol, sodium, or sugar. These comments are based on sound nutrition principles for weight loss or maintenance or management of diabetes, heart disease, and/or high blood pressure.

Managing the menu

This section, found in most chapters, provides specific suggestions about foods to order or avoid, depending on the type and category of restaurant. Suggestions are given for choosing appetizers, soups, main courses, side dishes, and even desserts.

The recommended choices are based on the nutrition modifications for a variety of medical conditions, from following a lower-sodium meal plan to reduce high blood pressure to reducing blood cholesterol through a low-fat and low-cholesterol diet.

Green Flag Words

The Green Flag Words provide you with a list of foods and preparation methods, typical of a particular style restaurant, that signal a go-ahead green light for ordering. These are the menu items, ingredients, or styles of preparation that are relatively low in fat, saturated fat, cholesterol, sodium, and calories compared to other dishes and styles of preparation you'll likely find on the menu. You will frequently see the words "steamed," "poached," "barbecued," and "grilled" on the list of Green Flag Words. It might be helpful to review the specific list of Green Flag Words prior to eating a particular fare so you can keep them in mind when reading the menu. Ordering these items will assist you in meeting your personal nutrition goals.

Red Flag Words

The Red Flag Words are words of caution, and they are intended to evoke thoughts of a stop sign. Red Flag Words indicate that those menu items, ingredients, and preparation methods should be avoided. Generally, these words deserve a red flag because they are high in fat, saturated fat, and/or cholesterol. It is probable that the calorie content of that item is also quite high. Usually fat and calories go hand-in-hand. A Red Flag Word might also point out an ingredient with too much sodium. Some Red Flag Words you'll find commonly listed are: "deep fried," "topped with melted cheese," "cheese sauce," and "heavy cream sauce." As you peruse the menu, look for the Red Flag Words and practice caution with these items when making your selections.

Special Requests

This section provides you with special requests that you can make when ordering a menu item in a particular type of restaurant. The special request might assist you in obtaining special preparation, eliminating a particular ingredient, or adding more of one food and leaving out another. These special requests are not intended to make dining out difficult or to ruffle any feathers. They are simple in nature and intended only to help you enjoy your food more in the knowledge that you are eating healthier or sticking closer to the specific recommendations of your special meal plan.

A commonly used special request when ordering a salad is, "May I have the salad dressing on the side?" When ordering a Mexican salad, you might ask, "Can the sour cream and/or guacamole be held or put on the side?" This obviously allows you to control the quantity used. You might ask to have a fish entree broiled "dry" or with margarine rather than butter. You might simply ask to have the fried, dry Chinese noodles removed from the table as you are seated. If you order a chef's salad, you might wish some of the egg and cheese to be exchanged for more turkey, roast beef, ham, or tuna. As you can see, once again, most of these special requests will assist you in limiting fat, saturated fat, cholesterol, and calories. The more often you make special requests when dining out, the more comfortable you will become practicing the strategy.

Typical menu

This section, included in most chapters, provides you with a typical menu for that particular type of restaurant. The items listed represent the gamut from best to worst choices that usually appear on that type of menu. Generally speaking, if you go into a Chinese restaurant in San Francisco, Chicago, or Miami, you will find similar menu listings. The same holds true for most ethnic cuisines. When considering fast food chains, however, you know only too well what menu choices to expect from coast to coast and beyond.

The "Typical Menu" is intended to provide you with a role-playing experience. Use it in advance to review the kinds of items you will see when the menu is placed in your hands as you sit down in the restaurant. This section gives you an opportunity to do some pre-planning. If you know you will be dining at a particular type of restaurant, open the book to that chapter and check out what's best to order for your specific needs.

We have used a small check mark in front of menu items that are "Preferred Choices." This simply means that we regard them as healthier choices than items not checked because they are lower in fat, cholesterol, or calories—the main factors to monitor when making food selections. In some cases a checked item should be eaten in moderation or modified according to directions in the "May I Take Your Order" section.

May I take your order

The final section in most restaurant chapters, "May I Take Your Order," provides you with "Model Meals," or ordering examples, based on different nutritional goals. The five examples given range from low calorie/low fat to higher calorie/low cholesterol to low sodium. The models are intended to provide realistic suggestions for what you should consider ordering when dining out at that particular kind of restaurant. The model meals will help you realize that eating out within the parameters of your desired health goals is easily done. You can enjoy tasty, satisfying menu selections no matter what kind of cuisine you have chosen.

The five model meals are numbered 1 to 5 simply for quick reference, are intended to cover a wide variety of dietary goals and are designed for people on special meal plans, for those simply trying to eat healthier, and for people maintaining their newly defined waistlines. The following provides a brief description of each model meal category. Look these over and try to match your nutrition goals with one of these categories. Then, prior to eating out, you will know which model to use as a guide.

❶ **Low Calorie/Low Fat:** These meals, on average, will contain approximately 400–700 calories, with 30–40% of the total calories from fat. They are based on a total daily intake in the range of 1,200–1,600 calories. If you are targeting toward the 1,200 calorie mark, observe the total calories of the meal. If you think it's too high, consider eliminating a food that will allow you to eat closer to your calorie target. There is an effort to strike a balance between encouraging you to try interesting and perhaps new taste treats and maintaining a focus on nutritional goals. The model meals are simply intended to meet generally accepted guidelines for achieving a low fat and low saturated fat diet. They will, in addition, be moderate to low in cholesterol and sodium.

These Low Calorie/Low Fat meals are quite appropriate for women and men attempting to lose weight as well as for women who are striving to maintain their present weight or newly achieved weight loss. The sample meals are also designed to meet the dietary recommendations of those with diabetes who have been encouraged to follow a meal plan in the range of 1,200–1,600 calories per day. These meals meet the American Diabetes Association's nutrition principles for meal planning. For this reason, desserts are often eliminated from these model meals. The "guestimated" exchange values that are provided are based on the 1986 Exchange Lists for Meal Planning developed by the American Diabetes Association and American Dietetic Association.

❷ Low Calorie/Low Cholesterol: These model meals can almost be used interchangeably with ones designated Low Calorie/Low Fat. However, these maintain more focus on keeping cholesterol content quite low: 100–200 mg per meal. The meals will contain an average of 400–700 calories and will be based on a daily total intake in the range of 1,200–1,600 calories. These meals will also generally be moderate to low in saturated fat and sodium. As always, in recommending these meals there is an effort to encourage adventure in dining and trying new and different taste treats that you might not have thought you could enjoy.

The Low Calorie/Low Cholesterol model meals are most appropriate for men and women with heart disease and/or elevated blood cholesterol who have been encouraged to decrease their body weight and to reduce their dietary cholesterol and saturated fat intake. These meals can also be used by those simply striving to maintain or achieve their desired body weight and/or eat in a healthier fashion.

❸ **Higher Calorie/Low Fat:** The model meals in this category total in the range of 600–1,000 calories. They are based on a total daily caloric intake between 1,800 and 2,200. These meals are designed to be low in fat; on average, only 30–40% of their total calories comes from fat. Generally speaking, these meals are also relatively moderate to low in saturated fat and cholesterol. They can be successfully utilized by large men who are attempting to lose weight. The meals are also appropriate for those wishing to maintain their present weight and for those simply interested in eating healthy. They are also intended to meet the nutrition principles for diabetes management, which is one reason why desserts have been eliminated. The sample meals are appropriate for those with diabetes who have been encouraged to follow a meal plan within the range of 1,800–2,200 calories per day. "Guestimated" exchange values for diabetes meal planning are provided.

❹ **Higher Calorie/Low Cholesterol:** These model meals can basically be used interchangeably with the Higher Cholesterol/Low Fat meals. These meals are in the range of 600–1,000 calories each. They are based on a total daily intake of 1,800–2,200 calories. The individual examples are designed to contain approximately 100–200 milligrams of cholesterol. They are generally moderate to low in saturated fat and sodium. These meals are intended to be used by individuals attempting to lower blood cholesterol levels by following American Heart Association dietary guidelines and by those simply trying to follow general nutritional recommendations for healthy eating and weight maintenance.

❺ **Low Sodium:** These model meals provide suggestions for those whose main dietary priority is to maintain a low sodium intake. The examples are designed to contain approximately 1,000–1,500 milligrams of sodium per meal, which nicely matches guidelines for maintaining low to moderate sodium intake. These meals are based on a total sodium intake average of 2,000–3,000 milligrams per day. For many people maintaining low sodium intake, this is simply one part of their dietary program, along with monitoring dietary cholesterol or fat. However, moderate to low sodium intake may be the only dietary restriction for some who have high blood pressure. Maintaining sodium consumption of approximately 3,000 milligrams per day or less is recommended for the general public.

Estimated Nutrient Evaluation: For each of the model meals you will find an estimated nutrient evaluation pertinent to that specific meal. Estimated total calories and percentage of calories from fat, protein, carbohydrates, and alcohol (if included in the meal) are given, along with cholesterol and sodium content. For reference, generally accepted nutrition goals for percentage of calories from fat, protein, and carbohydrates are shown, as are goals for cholesterol and sodium. The estimated nutrient evaluations are based on sample recipes and nutrient composition tables from the United States Department of Agriculture (USDA).

It is important to keep in mind that these are simply estimates. Figures are based on estimates of usual amounts of ingredients used in a menu item and the usual quantity served. As there are thousands of restaurants with thousands of cooks and chefs preparing food in different ways, it would be impossible to provide anything more defined than an "estimate." However, more and more chain restaurants, especially the fast food ones, are making the nutrient evaluation of their foods available upon request. Estimations in the Fast Food chapter are based on information provided by several of these companies.

Another important point to keep in mind when you are looking over the estimated nutrient evaluations is to think about fitting these meals into the context of your food intake for the entire day and week. For example, if you are on a low sodium dietary program and you know you will be having dinner out at a Chinese restaurant, you may wish to tightly restrict your sodium intake during the day, prior to dining out. This will, in essence, allow you to "bank" some of your sodium milligrams for your evening meal.

Now on to healthier eating out in virtually all kinds of restaurants.

4

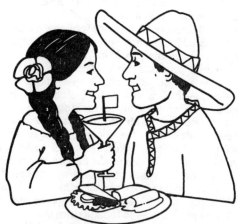

Healthier eating out
Mexican Style

I f you like foods hot, spicy, and loaded with
jalapeños peppers, Mexican food is probably
high on your list of ethnic cuisines enjoyed
when dining out. You're in sync with the rest
of the American public. Overall, the National
Restaurant Association names Mexican food as one
of the three most popular ethnic cuisines. However,
the healthiness of Mexican food might be of concern.
Memories of Mexican meals may conjure up thoughts
of high-fat nacho chips topped with high-fat guacamole and sour cream or of fried taco shells sprinkled
with high-cholesterol shredded cheese. Fortunately,

a Mexican meal has the potential of being quite healthy. Soft tacos filed with refried beans, lettuce, tomato, onions, and salsa; chicken enchiladas; or a Mexican salad are just a few of the great, healthier choices commonly available on Mexican menus.

Actually, many food aficionados say it's a misnomer to refer to the foods Americans call Mexican as truly Mexican. There are people who insist that chili con carne is an invention that originated in Texas, and one certainly would not find a "Mexican" salad in a crisp tortilla shell served in Mexican homes. Like most ethnic cuisines, there have been American adaptations and interpretations.

Some people refer to the foods we know as Mexican as Tex-Mex or Mexican-American. These recipes and concoctions have their roots in Mexican cooking, but the finished products don't identically match the dishes native to Mexico. Many of the basic ingredients—chilies, beans, and corn—remain the same, as well as some of the cooking methods.

To understand more about the roots of Mexican cuisine one needs to trace the history of Mexico. The basic origins of Mexican cookery hark back to Aztec and Mayan Indian civilizations, the early settlers of this territory. The foods they commonly ate still predominate in Mexico today—beans, corn, and tomatoes. In the 1500s the Spanish descended and spread their food habits and preferences to the Mexican culture. They introduced more protein in the form of pork, beef, and poultry. Other ingredients that became integrated into the cooking style of Mexico were garlic, cinnamon, onions, rice, and sugar. In addition to the Spanish, there were additional European influences in Mexican cuisine over the years. In fact, it is said the Germans are responsible for teaching the Mexicans how to brew beer.

Even though there seems to be a distinction made by some experts between Mexican and Tex-Mex food, there doesn't seem to be a tremendous difference. It's true that corn, beans, and chilies are basic to Mexican cuisine. Some say that beans are included in all Mexican meals. Preparation methods commonly used are frying, stewing, braising, and marinating. Obviously, these cooking methods reflect the lack of baking ovens in early times.

Few dairy products are included in the Mexican diet. Tortillas, made from corn, are often called the bread of Mexico. Tortillas can also be made from wheat. Many one-dish meals are served, such as stews. Mexican "breads" are typically stuffed with beef, pork, chicken, or cheese. Tacos, burritos, and enchiladas are examples of stuffed items. Originally, the beef, pork, or chicken was usually tough, so preparation methods of marinating, braising, or stewing were used to soften them. The coffee and cocoa bean are native and plentiful in Mexico. They are both, therefore, commonly served beverages.

Traditionally, Mexicans eat five meals each day. An early breakfast, called *desayuno,* consists of coffee or cocoa with a roll. *Almuerzo,* the second meal, is bigger and somewhat analogous to our brunch. Fruit, tortillas, eggs, and coffee are typically served. *Comida* is the main meal of the day, consumed in the afternoon. This meal can include up to six courses: appetizers, soup, chicken or fish, beans, dessert, and coffee. The last two light meals of the day are called *merienda* and *cena.*

The proximity of Mexico to the United States certainly influences the impact of Mexican cuisine on our culture. Actually, the states of Texas, New Mexico, Arizona, and parts of Colorado, Nevada, and California were part of Mexico prior to the 1800s. Unique to the United State's relationship with Mexico is the shared border of about two thousand of our southwestern miles. There has been and continues to be a large influx of Mexicans into the United States. The Mexican-American population, though dispersed throughout the country, is still predominantly in the Southwestern border states.

The large and growing Mexican population within the United States has certainly contributed to the ever-growing melting pot of foods available in supermarkets and American, as well as Mexican, restaurants. Consider the average supermarket today – it's usual to find chili con carne, tortillas, refried beans, chili powder, and other typically Mexican foods. It's also common to find Mexican foods integrated into American menus, for instance, chili burgers, nachos, and Mexican salads.

Today, more and more people are enjoying Mexican food, or what we'll more appropriately call Tex-Mex. Mexican restaurants are found in almost every city in the United States. However, you still find more Mexican eateries in the Southwestern region – Texas,

New Mexico, Arizona, and California. Mexican cooking in this part of the country is more authentic and traditional. There are more independently owned and operated establishments in the Southwest. I've lived about as far away from the Mexican border as one can and know first-hand that Mexican restaurants in the Northeast are for the most part popular chains. An independently owned Mexican restaurant here is a rarity.

In the United States today, Mexican food is found in a variety of eating establishments. There are many Mexican fast food stops where you're sure to find tacos, burritos, and enchiladas. There are numerous mid-price range Mexican food chains that feature nachos, tacos, enchiladas, chili con carne, and large Mexican salads. Mexican salads, nachos, hamburgers topped with chili, and chili con carne with chips have also found their way onto the menus of many American restaurants. The fast food and Mexican restaurant chains perhaps represent the greatest adulteration of true Mexican cuisine. On the upscale side, however, there are Mexican dining establishments serving entrees such as arroz con pollo, mole poblano, and pescado de Veracruz.

No matter whether it's authentic Mexican, Tex-Mex, or a Mexican salad or bowl of chili in an American restaurant, the taste of Mexican food packs lots of punch, a cuisine you definitely want to continue to enjoy. Though there are numerous items you'll want to steer clear of, there are also many healthy choices.

What to consider before ordering

Being successful at dining out healthy on Mexican food definitely requires some serious navigating around the menu. The three mainstay ingredients of Mexican cooking are the healthy carbohydrate-containing corn, beans, and chilies. These three items find their way into most Mexican meals. Corn, beans, and chilies on their own are nutritionally sound, but when incorporated into Mexican appetizers or entrees, they can result either in nutritional disasters or wise choices. For instance, chilies are used as a main ingredient in chili con queso, a high-fat, spicy cheese dip, and in salsa verde, a low-fat, hot green sauce. Corn or wheat is the main ingredient in tortillas. In a soft taco, the flour tortilla contains little fat, whereas taco shells are deep fried. So, once again, making the right choices, depending on your nutritional needs, is of prime importance.

Another health benefit of Mexican food is the minimal focus on the protein content of the meal compared with a typical American meal. Compare the small quantity of meat, one to two ounces, in one enchilada with an eight- to ten-ounce steak common on American menus. This has its roots in the old practice of making minimal protein feed many people.

Fat is (as always) the villain in Mexican cuisine. Not only are there many fried items but many Mexican recipes traditionally call for the use of lard or animal fat drippings. Both of these items contain cholesterol and saturated fat. With increasing emphasis on decreasing the use of animal fats, perhaps more vegetable oil will be used in restaurant food preparation in the near future.

You might want to ask the waitperson to find out what type of fat is used in the cooking, especially if this is a restaurant you frequent. This information might well assist you in making wise menu choices. For instance, you might choose a soft taco rather than a hard taco if you know that the shell will be fried in lard. If vegetable oil is used for frying, you might feel better about ordering the chicken or beef fajitas. If calories are your biggest concern, then any fat of any type should be avoided if possible.

Mexican food also has the potential to be high in sodium. Salt is used in many recipes, and a lot of the food preparation is done prior to placing your order, such as preparing meats to stuff into tacos or burritos. This makes it difficult to request that limited salt be used on your foods. However, if you are ordering a dish such as grilled chicken, fish, or beef in an upscale Mexican restaurant, you might be successful with a request to limit salt. Chips and salsa and large amounts of cheese can also contribute to raising the sodium level. However, even though salsa contains salt, it's not that much. Due to its zesty taste, small amounts of salsa can be used to add punch to salads or chicken and fish dishes. Green or red is fine to use in small amounts.

Managing the menu

Unfortunately, the first items that often greet you at your table without request are the addictive chips and salsa. The first basket is emptied before you know it, and the waiter will gladly provide refills. The corn tortilla chips are deep fried and often salted (to encourage sipping on margaritas or beer). You can exercise the utmost of willpower and promise yourself to limit the number you eat, or, easier yet, never let the basket reach your table in the first place. Hopefully, you have compassionate dining partners or ones with similar healthy eating goals in mind.

The salsa is the winning half of the chips and salsa. Salsa, either red or green, is basically made with tomatoes, onions, chilis, some spices, and salt. It is quite low in calories, has zero fat, and adds a lot of pizazz if the chili content is high.

After you deal with the chips and salsa, you will have the menu in hand and will likely observe the appetizer listings. There are some fine choices, but they lurk behind many high-fat, fried items. The healthier choices you might find are gazpacho, ceviche, a cup of chili con carne, or black bean soup. You know the ones to avoid—nachos, the fried tortilla chips with melted cheese and jalapeños, and super nachos, which adds insult to injury by loading on top of the chips and melted cheese, refried beans, sour cream, and guacamole along with lettuce and tomatoes. Chili con queso, guacamole and chips, or quesadillas are also nutritional disasters.

If your dining partners are ordering high-fat appetizers, think about starting with a cup of chili or a bowl of the frequently served black bean soup. You might want to start with a Mexican dinner salad to help take the edge off your appetite and prevent you from indulging in the undesirable appetizers. Remember to ask that the dressing be put on the side; or to make your salad more Mexican, ask for a side of salsa and use it as a zero-calorie salad dressing. I gave this suggestion to a friend of mine, and he started this practice at home as well as when out enjoying Mexican food.

Moving on to the main course, Mexican entrees frequently use chicken, beans, corn- or wheat-based breads, lettuce, tomatoes, onions, peppers, and chilies. These are all healthy ingredients on any meal plan. Be on the look out for some of them when making your selections. There are also many high-fat and high-calorie ingredients found in Mexican entrees, including cheese (often Monterey Jack), sour cream, chorizo (Mexican sausage), guacamole, fried tortilla shells, and chips.

Chicken or beef enchiladas, burritos, or soft tacos are great choices. Fajitas, which seem to have made their way into many American as well as Mexican restaurants, are a great choice. Often the choice of chicken, beef, or shrimp or a combination of all three is available. A bowl of chili con carne, hold the cheese but serve with plenty of onions, is a good order to which a salad makes a nice complement. A Mexican salad with either spicy beef or preferably chicken is a great selection, although it's best if the fried tortilla shell or chips can be omitted.

It's always smart to ask that several ingredients be minimized or deleted: sour cream, guacamole, cheese, and olives. At the more upscale restaurants you will likely find a chicken or seafood dish that is grilled or served with a spicy tomato sauce. Items to steer clear of due mainly to their fat content are chimichangas, flautas, and chilies rellenos.

In addition to the menu items you expect to find in a Mexican restaurant—tacos, enchiladas, and nachos—many menus feature unique appetizers, entrees, or desserts. Some Mexican restaurants and/or fast food chains have developed unique items that you will only find served in those establishments. For instance, one popular Mexican chain has an item they call "chajitas," which are described as marinated strips of chicken, steak, or pork presented in a skillet with onions, peppers, and tomatoes. These are served with flour tortillas and very much resemble fajitas. Some of these chains also make more seafood choices available than are usually found on Mexican menus. It is important to look beyond simply what you know is safe to eat and explore what each individual menu has to offer. There may be some good choices lurking in the fine print that will provide new taste treats.

Along with many Mexican dinners come the starches—Mexican rice and frijoles refritos, better known as refried beans. In some restaurants a side of black beans, plain white rice, or guacamole might be served. Beans (usually pinto or black) are high in carbohydrate and also contain some soluble fiber, which has been found to slightly lower cholesterol, triglycerides, and blood glucose levels. However, don't get too excited; the frequently served refried beans are often refried in lard. Black beans, a side order of Mexican rice, or a side order of soft flour tortillas are better choices.

Take advantage of the ability to order à la carte in most Mexican restaurants. This enables you to really pick and choose exactly what you want. Perhaps, if you are strictly watching your calories and fat intake, the dinner salad and a cup of chili will be enough, or maybe adding a chicken enchilada will complete your meal. You might wish to order one burrito and one enchilada and get a salad to help fill you up. It is probably best if the combination plates are avoided. For most people, this is simply too much food and includes too many foods that need to be avoided.

The list of desserts in Mexican restaurants is usually minimal. The most commonly known Mexican dessert is an absolute nutritional disaster—sopaipillas, or deep-fried bread. The closest relative to sopaipilas is an American favorite on the state fair trail: fried dough. Another familiar Mexican dessert found on the menus of more upscale restaurants is flan, a sort of custard. Not a bad choice compared to others. If cholesterol is a problem, flan is probably best traded off for a great cup of Mexican coffee or espresso.

When the menu arrives, look for certain key words and phrases that signal the nutritional advisability of the items. We call them "Green Flag" (go for it) and "Red Flag" (steer clear) words.

Green Flag Words

shredded spicy chicken
spicy beef
spicy ground beef
served with salsa (hot red tomato sauce)
served with salsa verde (green chili sauce)
covered with enchilada sauce
topped with shredded lettuce, diced tomatoes, and onions
served with or wrapped in a corn or flour tortilla
grilled
marinated
picante sauce
simmered
with chilies

vegetarian
tomato sauce
mole sauce

topped with sour cream
served with guacamole
topped, filled, covered with cheese
shredded cheese
served in fried tortilla shell
stuffed with Mexican cheese
Red Flag
Words
Mexican cheese sauce
bacon
chorizo (Mexican sausage)
served over tortilla chips
topped with black olives
crispy
fried
deep fried
layered with refried beans

Please hold the sour cream.
Please hold the guacamole.
Please serve my salad without the
    fried tortilla shell (or nacho
    chips) but bring an order of soft
    tortillas on the side.
Special
Requests
Mexican
Style
Please remove the chips and salsa
    from the table.
Please don't bring any chips and
    salsa.
Please hold the grated cheese.
Would it be possible to get extra
    salsa on the side?
Please put extra shredded lettuce,
    tomatoes, and chopped onions on
    the plate.
Would it be possible to substitute
    shredded spiced chicken for
    beef?
Could I get this wrapped up to
    take home?

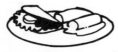

Typical Menu: Mexican Style

Appetizers ✓**Tostada** chips with hot salsa
Tostada chips with guacamole
Nachos served with melted
cheese and jalapeños peppers
Super nachos (fried tostado chips
with layers of beans and spicy
ground beef, covered with melted
cheese, and topped with lettuce,
tomato, onion, and sour cream)
Chili con queso (melted cheese,
green chilies, and peppers served
with corn tortilla chips)
✓**Black bean soup,** cup or bowl
✓**Chili con carne,** cup or bowl
✓**Gazpacho** (spicy cold soup made
from a blend of fresh vegetables
and tomatoes)

Salads ✓**Dinner salad** of mixed greens,
cheese, tomato, and bacon bits,
topped with onions
✓**Mexican salad** of lettuce, tomato,
and red peppers, topped with two
kinds of cheese, served in a crisp
tortilla shell, and served with
creamy garlic dressing
✓**Mexican chicken salad** of mixed
greens, diced tomatoes, and onions, topped with shredded spicy
chicken, shredded cheese, sliced
olives, and sour cream and
guacamole

✓*Preferred Choice*

✓**Taco salad**–a choice of spicy ground meat or shredded chicken, topped with refried beans, lettuce, tomatoes, and onions, topped with sour cream and guacamole and served in a crisp tortilla shell

Mexican Specialties Each item can be served à la carte or with refried beans and Mexican rice

Chimichangas, beef or chicken (flour tortillas filled with spicy beef or chicken and Monterey Jack cheese, fried and topped with tomato sauce)

✓**Fajitas** (marinated beef, chicken, or shrimp grilled with onions, green peppers, lettuce, diced tomatoes, sour cream, and guacamole)–single or double order for two available

✓**Enchiladas** (corn tortillas stuffed with either ground beef or shredded chicken and topped with tomato sauce and shredded cheese and served with sour cream)

✓**Tacos** (fried flour tortillas stuffed with your choice of spicy ground beef, shredded chicken, or a seafood blend; loaded with shredded lettuce, diced tomatoes, and onions and topped with cheese)

✓**Burritos** (large flour tortilla filled with a choice of refried beans and cheese, spicy ground beef, or chicken; served with tomato sauce and topped with shredded cheese)

Tostadas (crisp corn tortillas covered with black beans, chili verde, and choice of chicken or beef filling and topped with lettuce, tomato, and onions)

Mexican Dinners	Served with refried beans and Mexican rice

> **Flautas con crema** (crisp rolled tortillas stuffed wtih shredded chicken or beef, topped with a spicy cream sauce)
>
> ✓**Chili verde** (pork simmered with green chilies, vegetables, and Mexican spices)
>
> **Mole pollo** (boned chicken breast cooked in mole sauce, hot and spicy)
>
> ✓**Camarones de hacha** (fresh shrimp sauteed in a red and green tomato coriander sauce)
>
> **Carne asada** (grilled sirloin steak served in an enchilada sauce with chorizo and guacamole)
>
> ✓**Arroz con pollo** (boneless chicken breast served on top of spicy rice with vegetable sauce)

Side Orders	✓**Mexican rice** **Refried beans** ✓**Black beans** ✓**Tortillas,** flour or corn ✓**Salsa** **Guacamole**
Desserts	✓**Flan** (caramel-flavored custard) **Sopaipillas** (deep-fried dough, tossed in sugar)

Now that you've seen what may be available on the menu, look over the following five "Model Meals" for suggestions on how to order to achieve specific nutritional goals. Models are numbered one to five for quick reference, and each is followed by an "Estimated Nutrient Evaluation" that analyzes the content of that meal.

May I Take Your Order

Healthy	30% Calories as fat
Daily	20% Calories as protein
Eating	50% Calories as carbohydrate
Goals	300 mg/day Cholesterol
	3000 mg/day Sodium

❶

Low Calorie/	**Chili con carne**
Low Fat	*Quantity:* 1 cup
Model Meal	*Exchanges:* 1 starch; 1 meat; 1 fat
	Dinner salad (hold the cheese and dressing)
	Quantity: 2 cups
	Exchanges: 2 vegetable
	Salsa for dressing
	Exchanges: Free
	Chicken taco, soft
	Quantity: 1
	Exchanges: 1 starch; 2 meat; 1 fat

Estimated	480 calories
Nutrient	35% calories as fat
Evaluation	26% calories as protein
	39% calories as carbohydrate
	67 mg cholesterol
	1600 mg sodium

❷

Low Calorie/	**Dinner salad** (hold the cheese and dressing; use salsa)
Low	*Quantity:* 2 cups
Cholesterol	**Fajitas,** chicken and shrimp (hold the sour cream)
Model Meal	*Quantity:* 2 (1 oz. of chicken or shrimp in each)
	Mexican rice
	Quantity: ⅔ cup

Estimated	570 calories
Nutrient	25% calories as fat
Evaluation	26% calories as protein
	49% calories as carbohydrate
	120 mg cholesterol
	1100 mg sodium

❸
Higher Calorie/ Low Fat Model Meal

Black bean soup
Quantity: 1 cup
Exchanges: 2 starches
Chili verde served with 2 flour tortillas
Quantity: 1½ cups
Exchanges: 2 starch; 3 meat; 2 fat; 2 vegetable
Mexican rice
Quantity: ⅓ cup
Exchanges: 1 starch
Refried beans
Quantity: ⅓ cup
Exchanges: 1 starch; 1 fat
Mexican beer
Quantity: 12 oz

Estimated	992 calories
Nutrient	27% calories as fat
Evaluation	17% calories as protein
	48% calories as carbohydrate
	8% calories as alcohol
	96 mg cholesterol
	2100 mg sodium

❹
Higher Calorie/Low Cholesterol Model Meal

Tostada chips
Quantity: 10
Salsa
Quantity: 3 tbsp
*Burrito, bean and cheese
Quantity: 1
Chicken enchilada (hold cheese)
Quantity: 1
Mexican rice
Quantity: ⅓ cup
Black beans (request as substitute for refried beans)
Quantity: ⅓ cup
*Request extra lettuce and diced tomatoes, 1 cup

Estimated Nutrient Evaluation

780 calories
34% calories as fat
19% calories as protein
47% calories as carbohydrate
60 mg cholesterol
2000 mg sodium

❺
Low Sodium Model Meal

Mexican salad with shredded chicken, spicy black beans, lettuce, tomatoes, and onion
Quantity: 3–4 cups
Guacamole (on the side; hold the sour cream)
Quantity: ¼ cup
Salsa verde for dressing
Quantity: 4 tbsp
Corn tortillas
Quantity: 2
Flan (split order with friend)

Estimated	720 calories
Nutrient	31% calories as fat
Evaluation	28% calories as protein
	39% calories as carbohydrate
	197 mg cholesterol (125 from flan)
	950 mg sodium

Learn the terms of Mexican cuisine

Arroz–Spanish word for rice. Mexican rice is made from long-grain white rice with sauteed tomatoes, onions, and garlic added for flavor.

Burrito–a wheat flour tortilla (soft, not fried) filled with either chicken, beef, or cheese in addition to refried beans; served rolled up and covered with a light tomato-based enchilada sauce.

Carne–Spanish word for meat.

Cerveza–Spanish word for beer.

Ceviche–raw fish, soaked or "cooked" in lime or lemon juice for many hours and served as an appetizer or light meal; the seafood used is often scallops.

Chalupa–"little boat," a one-dish meal using corn meal topped with meat or chicken and beans and cheese.

Chili–there are over 100 different types of chilies native to Mexico. They are of different shapes, sizes, and colors, and they vary in level of spiciness from mild to hot, hotter, and hottest. Chilies are available fresh or dried.

Chili con carne–usually simply called "chili" in America, a thick soup made with tomatoes, onions, peppers, pinto beans, and ground or shredded beef; often served with raw chopped onions and shredded cheese.

Chimichanga–flour tortilla filled with beef, chicken, cheese, and/or beans; deep fried and served topped with tomato-based sauce

Chorizo–Mexican pork sausage, hot and highly seasoned.

Cilantro–leafy green herb with a strong flavor frequently used in Mexican cooking; also called coriander.

Enchiladas–corn tortillas dipped in enchilada sauce, lightly fried, and then filled with a choice of chicken, beef, or cheese and served topped with light tomato-based enchilada sauce.

Fajitas–sauteed chicken or beef served with sauteed onions and green peppers, shredded lettuce, tomatoes, and guacamole; served with flour tortillas. Usually you roll your own at the table.

Flan–baked custard with a caramel top; contains mainly sugar, eggs, and cream, whole or condensed milk.

Gazpacho–spicy, cold tomato-based soup that contains pureed or pieces of raw vegetables.

Guacamole–mashed avocado, onion, tomatoes, garlic, lemon juice, and spices; served as a topping, as a dip with chips, or on the side. Avocado is high in fat; approximately 80 calories per ¼ avocado, though the fat is mainly monounsaturated and contains no cholesterol.

Jalapeños chili–a type of chili often mistakenly referred to as a pepper. A very small, hot, green chili used to spice or top certain menu items.

Mole–refers to a "concoction," usually a spicy brown seasoning mixture for chicken or meats that contains a small amount of chocolate.

Quesadillas–flour tortillas filled with cheese and chili mixture; tortilla is rolled and then fried.

Refried beans–pinto beans that have been cooked and then refried in lard and seasoned with onions, garlic, and chili.

Salsa–hot red sauce made from tomatoes, onions, and chili; appears automatically on the table of most Mexican restaurants.

Salsa verde–very hot green sauce made from tomatillo, the Mexican green tomato, and other spices.

Taco–corn tortilla filled with meat or chicken, shredded cheese, lettuce, and tomatoes; usually the corn tortilla is fried in the shape of a "U". Soft taco is usually made with a flour tortilla and is not fried.

Tamale–spicy filling of either meat or chicken, surrounded by moist corn meal dough and wrapped in corn husks or banana leafs; they are then steamed.

Tortilla–the "bread" of Mexico, a very thin circle of dough made either from corn or flour; often corn tortillas are fried into taco shells or chips and served with salsa.

Tostadas–crisp, deep-fried tortilla chips, or the whole fried tortilla, which then may be covered with various toppings such as cheese, beans, lettuce, tomato, and/or onions.

5

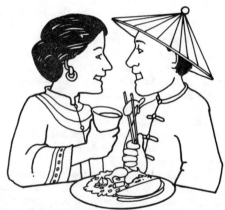

Healthier eating out
Chinese Style

C hinese food has become one of the most popular ethnic cuisines Americans enjoy when dining out. Chinese foods, markets, and cookery were virtually unknown in America prior to the mid-1800s. Today, it's commonplace to find at least several Chinese restaurants in most American cities. Now, beyond simply Cantonese-style cuisine, there are restaurants that specialize in the cuisines of different regions of China—Szechuan, Hunan, and Beijing. There's certainly more than just egg rolls, chop suey, pork-fried rice, and fortune cookies served in America's Chinese restaurants of the 1990s.

It was not until the mid-1800s that people from China began emigrating to the United States. During the later 1800s thousands of Chinese arrived. Many settled on the West Coast, many in California. These original Chinese settlers came from Canton. That's why Americans were and continue to be most familiar with Cantonese cuisine.

It was not until after World War II that another large influx of Chinese came to the United States. At that time people came from regions other than just Canton. There are now close to a million individuals of Chinese origin in America. Today, there are many native-born Chinese Americans as well.

Initially, when people from China came to the United States, it was common for them to settle in enclaves that became known as "Chinatown." Chinatowns developed in several large coastal cities—Boston, New York, San Francisco. These areas still thrive as social and cultural centers for people of Chinese origin. And the many Chinatowns across the country are still locales for little Chinese markets with fresh foods and Chinese specialty items. It's also true that some of the best Chinese food is found within the borders of Chinatowns. The specialty of the house might not be glamorous dining, but it often is great-tasting Chinese food.

There is a wide assortment of foods regularly used in Chinese cooking. Many of these foods are common to Americans, such as shrimp, chicken, broccoli, and sprouts. Yet there are others that, if you cook Chinese at home, you have to go to a Chinese market to purchase, such as lily buds and wood ears.

As is true for the origins of many ancient cuisines, a purpose can be traced for both the style of cookng and the ingredients used. For instance, stir-frying, the most common cooking method, was initially used because it was a means of cooking that conserved fuel. All foods were cut into small pieces, everything was cooked quickly, and minimal fuel was used. The reason why we see such odd items as wood ears, bamboo shoots, and lily buds is because the Chinese were resourceful. Food was not plentiful, and so just about anything became part of the diet.

Though almost all foods are included in Chinese cookery, it is not common to see dairy products used. That is true of many Asian cuisines. Rice is considered the staple of southern China, whereas northern

China is better known for wheat products. In American Chinese restaurants it's usual to see both rice and noodle dishes listed on the menu. Seafoods and animal protein sources—beef, pork, chicken, and duck—are seen everywhere in China. Soybeans are used to create a whole array of products from tofu (bean curd) to black bean sauce to the soy sauces that are integral to Chinese cooking.

Interestingly, little food in China is served raw, and salads are almost non-existent. Dishes might be cooked and then served cold, but we are most familiar with Chinese foods that are served hot. All of the appetizers we're familiar with are served hot.

Regional variations in Chinese cuisine

Americans are most accustomed to eating foods prepared in the Cantonese style. However, in the recent past there has been an increase in the number of Chinese restaurants serving Szechuan, Hunan, and Peking (Beijing) style cuisines. There is varying opinion from different experts as to whether there are three, four, or five regional cuisines of China. In reality, there are actually many more if one would delve into the many subtle regional differences. We will describe four seemingly distinct regional cooking styles. Many times, dishes on a Chinese menu will be named for that particular region; consider Peking duck, Szechuan spicy chicken, and Hunan crispy beef.

Canton is in the south of China. Cantonese dishes are often stir-fried, using mild and subtle flavors. Black bean and oyster sauce are commonly used. Seafood and pork are prevalent. Rice and soybeans are staples in this area of China and therefore became staples in Cantonese cooking. American Chinese restaurants still reflect the predominance of Canton's cooking techniques.

Moving to the northern regions of China, you find Beijing (Peking), Shantung (Shandong), and Honan (not Hunan) styles of cooking. Northern Chinese cooking styles were originally prepared for the palates of select citizens. Shantung has been defined as the "haute cuisine" of Chinese cooking. Beijing dishes were served at the ancient imperial court in Peking. Even today Peking duck is considered a very special item on Chinese menus. It is common to see sweet and sour sauces and plum or hoisin sauces used. Goodly amounts of onions and garlic are also familiar trademarks of northern cooking.

The western region is the home of hot and spicy Chinese cookery. This is Szechuan and Hunan style cuisine. Chilies, garlic, and hot red peppers (which you never want to bite into whole) are frequently used in this region. On Chinese menus in America, dishes from this region are often denoted in red. This distinguishes their hot and spicy nature. Interestingly, there are some broad similarities between Szechuan-style cuisine and the cooking of Thailand and Burma, neighbors to the south.

Probably the least familiar regional Chinese cooking style to Americans is that of Shanghai. Shanghai is in the eastern part of China. There, braising is a common preparation method. A combination of soy sauces, wine, and sugar is common to this region's cuisine. It is sometimes referred to as "red"cooking due to the braising process.

Chinese restaurants in America

Chinese restaurants in America occupy a broad range, from quick meal spots to elegant dining establishments. There are now even Chinese fast food stops. These are often found in large mall eatery sections. The Chinese fast food menu is usually limited to egg rolls, spare ribs, fried rice, sweet-and-sour dishes, chow mein, and a few other basically American inventions. The greatest number of Chinese restaurants are mid-price range and not very fancy. But there are also upscale Chinese restaurants whose table settings and service are truly elegant. Obviously, these extras are reflected in the price, but more luxurious Chinese restaurants are on the increase.

As is often true for ethnic cuisines in America, there are differences between the way food is typically served in America and protocols observed in China. Also, there are some foods that are not served at all in the U.S. due to lack of availability or limited popularity. In American Chinese restaurants you are often greeted with a bowl of fried noodles and then asked if you want something to drink, to which you might respond green tea, Tsing Tsao beer, or Planters Punch. Next, soup and/or appetizers are served, then come the entrees with rice, noodles, or both. Often pineapple and fortune cookies finish off a Chinese meal.

In China it is customary to serve most foods at the same time. If you have ever been at a Chinese restaurant late enough or have poked your head into the kitchen, you've probably observed the way Chinese ordinarily eat. The main dishes are placed in the center of the table, all for sharing. Each person has an individual bowl of white rice, which becomes a brief stopping place for food traveling from common bowls to private mouth. The place setting also includes chopsticks, a porcelain spoon for soup, a cup for wine or tea, and a small plate for bones. Lots of rice is consumed along with minimal amounts of protein and fat from the soup and entrees.

Whether it be Cantonese, Szechuan, or Shanghai, Chinese food eaten American style can either be a health-conscious eater's nightmare or a dream come true. It all depends on what you order and how much you consume. Consider the high fat, cholesterol, and sodium order of fried jumbo shrimps, egg drop soup, spicy beef with peanuts and scallions, and pork-fried rice. Conversely, picture the lower fat, cholesterol, and sodium order of steamed Peking raviolis, stir-fried sliced chicken with vegetables, and steamed white rice. There are multiple choices to be made in any Chinese restaurant no matter what your nutritional goals.

What to consider before ordering

Chinese food as it's eaten in China is healthier than it is in America. That is simply because the main focus for Americans, as usual, is on the protein portion of the meal, whereas in China the main focus is on the carbohydrates—white rice or noodles. Keep this in mind when you're eating a Chinese meal. Keep your focus on the carbos—the starches, vegetables, and fruits.

A Chinese meal can easily match the nutrition goals recommended for everyone's improved health, that is, higher carbohydrates and less protein, fat, and sodium. In addition, Chinese food certainly has the potential to be low in saturated fat and cholesterol. Rice and noodles are both mainly carbohydrate foods. Vegetables, also primarily carbohydrate, are abundant in Chinese cooking. There are many vegetables used that you are familiar with, such as broccoli, celery, carrots, and cabbage, and others that you may be less familiar with, such as bok choy, napa, wood ears, and lily buds (see "Learn the Terms of Chinese Cuisine" at the end of the chapter).

Fat is again one of the villains of Chinese cookery, but it is easy enough to pick and choose. If necessary, it's easy to make special requests to limit the fatty foods and added oils or high sodium sauces used in cooking. Remember, most dishes are prepared to order.

Several foods, such as duck, beef, and pork, which are higher in fat, can be limited. Many high-fat cuts of pork are used in Chinese cooking: spare ribs, for example. However, think of the frequently available roast pork strips appetizer. This pork is actually quite lean. The biggest problem with fat is the extra fat incorporated in cooking. There are many menu items, such as sweet-and-sour dishes, that are breaded and deep-fried and should consistently be avoided. There are also several Chinese appetizers that are deep-fried and should be avoided, namely eggrolls, fried shrimp, and fried won tons.

The most common cooking method used is stir-frying in a wok. In fact, it used to be rare to find an oven in China. A wok can also be used for methods of cooking other than stir-frying, such as braising and steaming. Cooking in a wok can actually be quite healthy. A minimal amount of oil can be used, and foods are cooked very briefly so they retain their vitamin and mineral content.

Traditionally, much lard (pork fat) was used in Chinese cooking, but according to some, more liquid oil is used today. Peanut oil is commonly used due to its high smoking point. Peanut oil also casts a slightly nutty flavor to dishes. It's mainly a monounsaturated fat, now thought to help lower blood cholesterol. Sesame seed oil is also used, but in smaller quantities. Sesame seed oil is a polyunsaturated fat, which also assists in lowering blood cholesterol. So, although oil used in Chinese cooking can be plentiful, the oils are healthy ones.

One other villain is the high sodium content of Chinese food. Many dishes contain both the high-sodium soy sauces, light and dark, and MSG (monosodium glutamate). Other sauces such as oyster, black bean, and hoisin also contain large amounts of sodium. For frame of reference, a tablespoon of soy sauce has about 1,000 milligrams of sodium and recommended daily intake is 3,000! Once again, there are ways to work around the high sodium content. However, Chinese food might not be the optimal choice, at least on a frequent basis, for individuals on a severely restricted sodium regimen.

To limit your sodium consumption, stay away from Chinese soups. Maybe you can find an appropriate appetizer or else jump right into the entrees. Steamed white rice is definitely a better choice than fried rice or one of the lo mein dishes, both of which have soy sauce added. Dishes with a lighter sauce, both in color and consistency, tend to have a lower sodium content than those with heavier sauces, such as hoisin, oyster, or black bean sauce.

There are some special requests you can make to decrease the sodium. Let the waitperson know you are concerned about salt, and ask him or her to pass that along to the chef. You can request that less soy and no MSG be used in your foods. Don't forget, all Chinese entrees are prepared to order, so special requests should be easy. I would not recommend saying no soy because the end product simply will be untasty. Think about using the sweet sauce, "duck" sauce, and hot mustard as low-sodium flavorings.

There are some facts about Chinese cooking of which people with diabetes should be aware. Surprisingly to some, there is sugar used in many Chinese dishes. Most times it's good old granulated white, and other times it's brown sugar. Some sauces are sweeter, such as hoisin sauce. Hoisin sauce commonly comes on the side with an order of moo shi. On average, a dish has in the range of a teaspoon to a tablespoon of sugar added to a recipe for 4–6 servings. When you divide that small amount into numerous servings, you realize that you get only a small amount: probably less than a half-teaspoon.

Chinese food certainly doesn't need to be avoided by people with diabetes, but you should be aware that sugar will regularly be used. One consideration for people who have diabetes is the sweet sauce that is placed on the table. This sauce should be avoided, at least in any volume. You might wish to request that sugar be left out of your dishes if you feel your blood sugar rises when you consume Chinese food. Howwever, you might be told that it is already premixed into marinades or sauces.

Interestingly, the rules about using some sugar in the diabetes meal plan have relaxed somewhat in the recent past. There was an article in *Diabetes Forecast*,

June, 1989, entitled "Relaxing the Rules," authored by Marion Franz, M.S.,R.D. It stated that the American Diabetes Association's rule of thumb for allowing a recipe to be printed is that it contain no more then one teaspoon per serving of sugar, honey, molasses, or other caloric sweetener. The previous guideline was less than one-half teaspoon.

Managing the menu

Many Chinese appetizers are simply off-limits if you're monitoring the fats. Consider fried shrimp, fried won ton, fried chicken, fried Peking raviolis. They all have that evil "F" word attached—fried. There are some appetizers to consider ordering: steamed Peking raviolis, roast pork strips, teriyaki beef or chicken (if sodium is not a big concern). Interestingly, many of the well known "Chinese" appetizers are really American inventions.

You might be best off skipping the high-fat appetizers and having a bowl of soup instead. You can order most soups individually although some are available only for two or more. So if your dining companions are indulging in appetizers, order a bowl of filling, low-calorie soup. This has the added benefit of decreasing your appetite when the entrees arrive. Hot-and-sour soup, sizzling rice soup with chicken or shrimp, Chinese vegetable, or delights of three are all acceptable alternatives. Note that soup will be high in sodium if that's a concern.

Among the entrees you will find many healthy choices. As many regions of China are near the ocean, a good deal of seafood is commonly used—shrimp, prawns, scallops, and fin fish. Other healthy protein foods frequently available are chicken and tofu (bean curd). When perusing the menu, look for dishes that contain vegetables. Which of these two descriptions sounds healthier: General Gau's chicken—cubes of chicken coated with water chestnut flour and eggs, deep fried until crispy, and then dry cooked with hot ginger sauce; or Moo Goo Gai Pan—sliced tender chicken meat sauteed with sliced water chestnuts, mushrooms, and Chinese mixed greens? Obviously, the second listing is better. Consider ordering dishes from the vegetable listings such as spicy green beans, broccoli in oyster sauce, or a vegetarian delight. This cuts down on protein and provides lots of filling, high-volume vegetables.

It's best to avoid the sweet-and-sour dishes, diabetes or not. The meat, chicken or pork, is always battered and fried before the heavy sweet sauce is added. Try to stay away from dishes that have nuts added—chicken and cashews or peanuts, for instance. They often do not include vegetables. Duck dishes can be higher in fat than you wish due to the high fat content of duck itself, especially the skin. Avoid Peking duck and crispy duck with plum sauce.

On to the starches—rice and noodles. Both seem always to be available in several different varieties, some healthy and some not. Obviously, white rice is best. It is steamed with no added salt or fats. Fried rice has additional fat and soy sauce added. If you order fried rice, stick with the vegetable-fried variety and avoid having more fat added in the form of pork or beef. Similar information holds true for lo mein. The basic noodle is quite healthy, but then oils and high-sodium sauces are added. If you order lo mein, have the vegetable or shrimp and avoid the pork and beef combinations. It's best to avoid the pan-fried noodles found on some menus. Lo mein is a better choice if you want noodles.

Dessert in Chinese restaurants is relatively underplayed. Often you don't even order it; pineapple, fortune cookies, and toothpicks simply arrive at your table. The limited listing of desserts usually includes pineapple chunks, lychee nuts, and ice cream. The pineapple or lychee nuts are fine choices. You'll leave the table healthier if you read the fortune and leave the cookie; fortune cookies just aren't usually worth the calories.

Chopsticks are the usual eating utensils of the Chinese, though forks and spoons are routinely made available to those unadept at using the sticks. If you're not good at using chopsticks, it might be a blessing in disguise. Your lack of dexterity will help slow down your pace of eating, so go ahead and be daring!

No matter which Chinese restaurant you choose, you probably will have a good sense of what you will find on the menu before it's placed in front of you. Therefore, before you even arrive at the restaurant, give some thought to what you might order. It is helpful to have some ideas in mind so your taste buds don't have a chance to do too much fantasizing. It's very common to share Chinese selections among eating partners. If that is the style in which you are ordering, be clear about your personal nutritional goals.

Make sure that foods are chosen that fit your plan.

Be careful to monitor your point of fullness and not overeat. Chinese restaurants are almost always equipped to make taking leftovers home easy. Think about how nice it will be to eat this or that food again for lunch or dinner the next day.

When the menu arrives, look for certain key words and phrases that signal the nutritional advisability of the items. We call them "Green Flag" (go for it) and "Red Flag" (steer clear) words.

Green Flag Words

lobster sauce
cooked in light wine sauce
simmered
steamed
roasted
bean curd (tofu)
with assorted vegetables: broccoli, mushrooms, onion, cabbage
stir-fried in mild sauce
hot and spicy tomato sauce
served on a sizzling platter
in slippery light sauce or velvet sauce
garnished with spinach or broccoli
fresh fish fillets

Red Flag Words

fried
deep fried
breaded and fried
deep fried until crispy
duck
hoisin sauce
with cashews or peanuts
pieces of egg
egg foo young
coated with water chestnut flour and fried
crispy (usually means breaded and fried)

dipped in batter and browned in
  oil
served with a rich sweet sauce
sweet-and-sour sauce
served in bird's nest
with plum sauce
soy sauce

**Special
Requests
Chinese
Style**

Please don't use MSG.

What type of oil is used for stir-
frying? (If lard or other saturated fat, request that peanut or
other available non-animal fat
be used.)

Would it be possible to use less oil
in the preparation?

Would it be possible to use less
salt and soy sauce?

Can you substitute chicken in this
dish for duck?

Could you substitute (or add in
more) broccoli and leave out the
spinach?

Please don't garnish with peanuts
or cashews.

Can you leave off the crispy fried
won ton?

Please remove the crispy fried
noodles from the table.

Typical Menu: Chinese Style

Appetizers   **Egg rolls** (2)
Spring rolls (2)
✓**Steamed Peking raviolis** (6)
Peking raviolis (6)
✓**Roast pork** strips
Barbecued spare ribs
✓**Teriyaki** beef or chicken on
skewers
Jumbo shrimp, fried
Won tons, fried
Pu pu platter for two—contains
egg rolls, spare ribs, fried shrimp,
and teriyaki beef

Soups   ✓**Hot-and-sour** soup
✓**Won ton** soup
✓**Sizzling** rice and chicken soup
✓**Sizzling** rice and shrimp soup
✓**Delights of three** (assorted Chi-
nese vegetables and chicken, pork,
and beef strips)
Egg drop soup

Poultry   ✓**Velvet chicken** (breast of
chicken, snow peas, water chest-
nuts, bamboo shoots, and a garnish of egg white)
*****General Gau's chicken** (cubes of
chicken coated with water-
chestnut flour and eggs, deep
fried until crispy, and coated with
hot ginger sauce)
Sweet-and-sour chicken
(chicken pieces battered and fried,
topped with a thick sweet-and-
pungent sauce, topped with
pineapples)

✓*Preferred Choice*

✓***Hunan spicy chicken** (spicy chicken with assorted vegetables)

✓**Chicken chop suey** (breast of chicken stir-fried with celery, Chinese cabbage, and other assorted vegetables)

Sweet-and-pungent duck (cubes of duck, dipped in batter, deep fried, and served with water chestnuts, cherries, and peas)

✓**Sizzling sliced chicken** with vegetables (sliced breast of chicken with assorted Chinese vegetables, served on a sizzling platter)

✓***Yu Hsiang chicken** (Strips of chicken stir-fried with bamboo shoots, water chestnuts, wood ears, lily buds, and Chinese cabbage)

Seafood ✓***Shrimp with tomato sauce** (shrimp sauteed with fine-diced bamboo shoots and scallions, mixed in a hot and spicy tomato sauce)

✓**Shrimp with broccoli** and mushrooms (stir-fried shrimp with broccoli and Chinese mushrooms in light egg white sauce)

***Spicy crispy whole fish** (a whole fish deep fried and coated with a hot, spicy sauce)

Shrimp and cashews (whole shrimp stir-fried with cashew nuts and water chestnuts)

✓***Szechuan** style fresh fish fillets (fish fillets sauteed with bamboo shoots and scallions, served with a hot and spicy sauce)

✓**Moo shi shrimp** (stir-fried shrimp with Chinese vegetables, served with Chinese pancakes and hoisin sauce)

Meats ✓**Beef and broccoli** with black
mushrooms (strips of beef sauteed
with broccoli and black
mushrooms in oyster sauce)
***Szechuan orange beef** (beef
coated with orange-flavored spicy
sauce)
✓***Twice cooked pork** (pork with
cabbage, green peppers, and bamboo shoots in hot bean sauce)
***Hunan crispy beef** (beef deep
fried and coated with a hot Hunan sauce, served surrounded by
broccoli)
✓**Sizzling lamb** (lamb and vegetables in a light sauce, served on a
sizzling platter)
✓**Roast pork** with vegetables
(slices of pork stir-fried with assorted Chinese vegetables)
✓**Beef chow mein** (sliced beef stir-
fried with diced cabbage, onions,
sliced mushrooms, and other Chinese vegetables)

Vegetables ✓**Vegetarian delight** (ten kinds of
crunchy vegetables stir-fried in a
light sauce)
***Yu Hsiang eggplant** (eggplant
stir-fried with other Chinese
vegetables)
✓***Spicy green beans** (green beans
sauteed in hot and spicy Hunan
sauce)
✓**Broccoli** and black mushrooms in
oyster sauce (broccoli and
mushrooms stir-fried with oyster
sauce and topped with peanuts)

*Indicates a hot and spicy dish.

Rice ✓**Steamed white rice** (small or
large bowl)
Beef-fried rice
Pork-fried rice

          ✓**Vegetable-fried rice**
          House special fried rice

Noodles   **Roast pork lo mein**
          ✓**Chicken lo mein**
          ✓**Vegetable lo mein**
          Pan-fried noodles with shrimp,
          pork, and chicken
          Pan-fried noodles with assorted
          Chinese vegetables

Desserts   ✓**Pineapple chunks**
          ✓**Lychee nuts**
          Vanilla ice cream
          Fried bananas served with sweet
          syrup sauce
          Fortune cookies

Now that you've seen what may be available on the menu, look over the following five "Model Meals" for suggestions on how to order to achieve specific nutritional goals. Models are numbered one to five for quick reference, and each is followed by an "Estimated Nutrient Evaluation" that analyzes the content of that meal.

May I Take Your Order

**Healthy
Daily
Eating
Goals**

30% Calories as fat
20% Calories as protein
50% Calories as carbohydrate
300 mg/day Cholesterol
3000 mg/day Sodium

**❶
Low Calorie/
Low Fat
Model Meal**

Hot-and-sour soup
Quantity: 1 cup
Exchanges: 1 vegetable
Yu Hsiang chicken
Quantity: 1½ cups (split order)
Exchanges: 2 meat; 1 fat; 1
  vegetable
Shrimp with broccoli and
  mushrooms
Quantity: 1 cup
Exchanges: 2 meat; 1 fat; 1
  vegetable
Steamed white rice
Quantity: ⅔ cup
Exchanges: 2 starch
Fortune cookie
(Read fortune; skip cookie)

**Estimated
Nutrient
Evaluation**

570 calories
35% calories as fat
29% calories as protein
36% calories as carbohydrate
150 mg cholesterol
1300 mg sodium+

❷

Low Calorie/ Low Cholesterol Model Meal	**Beef with broccoli** and black mushrooms *Quantity:* 1 cup (split order) **Vegetarian delight** *Quantity:* 1½ cups **Steamed white rice** *Quantity:* ⅔ cup **Lychee nuts** Quantity: ½ cup
Estimated Nutrient Evaluation	590 calories 38% calories as fat 22% calories as protein 40% calories as carbohydrate 52 mg cholesterol 915 mg sodium

❸

Higher Calorie/Low Fat Model Meal	**Peking raviolis,** steamed *Quantity:* 2 *Exchanges:* 1 starch; 1 meat; 1 fat; ½ vegetable **Moo shi shrimp** *Quantity:* 2 pancakes; 1½ cups filling (split order) *Exchanges:* 1 starch; 2 meats; 1 fat; 2 vegetable **Vegetable lo mein** noodles *Quantity:* 1½ cups (split order) *Exchanges:* 3 starch; 1 fat; 1 vegetable **Tsing Tsao beer** *Quantity:* 12 oz *Exchanges:* 1 starch; 1 fat

Estimated	911 calories
Nutrient	24% calories as fat
Evaluation	19% calories as protein
	49% calories as carbohydrate
	8% calories as alcohol
	134 mg cholesterol
	1300 mg sodium+

❹

Higher	**Sizzling rice** and chicken soup
Calorie/Low	*Quantity:* 1 cup
Cholesterol	**Velvet chicken**
Model Meal	*Quantity:* 1½ cups (split order)
	Szechuan fresh fish fillets
	Quantity: 1½ cups
	Vegetable-fried rice
	Quantity: 1 cup
	Pineapple
	Quantity: ½ cup

Estimated	687 calories
Nutrient	30% calories as fat
Evaluation	25% calories as protein
	45% calories as carbohydrate
	110 mg cholesterol
	1700 mg sodium+

❺

*Low Sodium	**Peking raviolis,** steamed (use
Model Meal	sweet sauce and mustard)
	Quantity: 2
	Sizzling sliced chicken with
	vegetables
	Quantity: 1½ cups (split order)
	Beef chow mein
	Quantity: 1½ cups
	Steamed white rice
	Quantity: ⅔ cup
	*Request that no MSG and less
	soy sauce be used.

Estimated	814 calories
Nutrient	37% calories as fat
Evaluation	25% calories as protein
	38% calories as carbohydrate
	135 mg cholesterol
	1200 mg sodium+

+Sodium values are based on usual preparation
methods determined from several Chinese cook-
books. If no MSG and less soy and other sauces
are requested, sodium intake can easily be
lowered.

Learn the terms of Chinese cuisine

Bean curd—known as "tofu" to Americans; made
from soy beans and formed into blocks; used
sliced or cubed in soups or dishes.

Black bean sauce—a thick, brown sauce made of
fermented soy beans, salt, and wheat flour; frequently used in Cantonese cooking.

Bok choy—looks like a cross between celery and
cabbage; also known as Chinese chard.

Five-spice powder—a reddish-brown powder,
combining star anise, fennel, cinnamon, cloves,
and Szechuan pepper; used in Szechuan dishes.

Hoisin sauce—a sweet and spicy thick sauce made
from soy beans, sugar, garlic, chili, and vinegar.

Lily buds—dried, golden-colored buds with a light,
flowery flavor; also called lotus buds and tiger
lily buds; used in entrees and soups.

Lychees—crimson-colored fruit with translucent
flesh around a brown seed, closely resembling a
white grape.

Monosodium glutamate (MSG)—a white powder
used in small amounts to bring out and enhance
the flavors of ingredients.

Napa—also referred to as Chinese cabbage, it has
thick-ribbed stalks and crinkled leaves.

Oyster sauce—a rich, thick sauce made of oysters,
their cooking liquid, and soy sauce; frequently
used in Cantonese dishes.

Plum sauce—an amber-colored, thick sauce made from plums, apricots, hot peppers, vinegar, and sugar, it has a spicy sweet-and-sour flavor; found on the table in many Chinese restaurants.

Sesame seed oil—oil extracted from sesame seeds, it has a strong sesame seed flavor and is used as seasoning for soups, seafood, and other dishes.

Soy sauce—either light or dark, used in virtually all Chinese dishes. Light soy tends to be used with poultry and seafoods.

Sweet-and-sour sauce—thick sauce made from sugar, vinegar, and soy sauce. Meat, chicken, or shrimp served with this sauce is usually dipped in batter and fried.

Wood ear—a variety of tree lichen, which is brown and resembles a wrinkled ear; it is soaked before use.

6

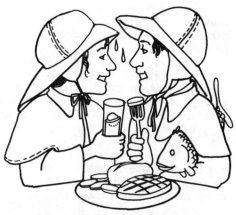

Healthier eating out
Seafood Style

Seafood, from fin fish to shellfish, is served in a wide range of restaurants and prepared in a multitude of different ways—from very healthy to decadently high in fat and cholesterol. Consider the broad difference between grilled swordfish and lobster Newburg. Seafood is found in restaurants solely dedicated to preparing only the freshest of seafood to surf and turf places, fine dining establishments, moderately priced family restaurants, and fast food spots specializing in quick, fried fish 'n chips or fried clams.

The message is loud and clear—eat more seafood: it's good for you. Indeed, the benefits of eating fish, once thought to be "brain food," are now confirmed by sound scientific data. And many Americans, knowing that fish is good for the heart as well as the waistline, have responded by consuming more seafood. Today's greater demand for seafood has been met by the restaurant industry through accessing and serving a wider variety of seafood choices and by simply having more seafood items on menus. In addition, more specialty seafood restaurants have sprouted up in response.

Due to modern transportation methods, restaurants can purchase and serve fresh fish almost anywhere in the country. Certainly, frozen fin fish and shellfish continue to be used in some, usually more moderately priced restaurants and in the fast food industry. And you still expect to see more seafood served in coastal cities, where it's more readily available.

It's common to find particular seafoods on menus in specific regions. For instance, Maryland offers soft shell crabs, and Alaska is known for its king crab. In Florida you find grouper, whereas up in the northwest corner of the United States there's plenty of salmon. And in New Orleans you're bound to be surrounded by tiny crayfish. But thanks to modern transportation, refrigeration, and consumer demand, you are now able to enjoy Maine lobster in Kansas City and yellowfin tuna, native to Hawaii, in Virginia. In fact, Legal Sea Foods, the well-known chain of seafood restaurants in Massachusetts, makes available the "Maine Event" by phone. This is a New England style clam bake that can be delivered, thanks to overnight shipping services, to your doorstep almost anywhere in the U.S. within 24 hours of placing your phone order.

There are many people who simply never eat seafood. In fact, there is a segment of the population that is allergic to fish. Some people are allergic to all types of fish, some just to shellfish. Others simply dislike fish and remain unadventurous about exploring the menu's seafood options. One important aspect of enjoying seafood is the importance of serving it extremely fresh. The shorter the time between catching and eating, the fresher and better tasting the fish. Of course, there are definitely some fish that, simply put, are "fishier," such as bluefish, fresh tuna, and mackeral. People who are squeamish about eating fish should be sure they are sampling it in a restaurant that concentrates on freshness. In addition, the less-than-enthusiastic should choose fish that is light in taste and consistency, such as flounder, sole, or scrod (which is really cod or haddock).

It might be said that the more you really enjoy the taste of fish, the more simply you like it prepared. If you don't really like fish, you might be tempted to cover up the flavor with lots of high-fat ingredients such as butter, cream sauces, and cheesy bread-crumbs. In general, seafood is relatively light in taste and therefore lends itself to a variety of different herbs, spices, and seasonings as well as many different cooking methods.

Due to increased desire by the public for more healthfully prepared fin fish and shellfish, many new and tasty cooking methods are now being used. Methods of grilling, possibly on mesquite chips, and blackening have come into vogue. Mustard sauces are used more often, along with simple lemon or wine sauces, garlic, and roasted pepper or spicy tomato salsa. All of these preparation methods add few calories and minimal fat and cholesterol to the end product.

What to consider before ordering

There are numerous reasons to eat more fish, from its low calorie count to its moderate cholesterol and low saturated fat content. All seafood, prior to preparation, is among the healthiest protein food available. But many of the health characteristics of fish can quickly be destroyed if it is prepared in a high-fat and high-calorie recipe. Consider the nutritional differences between a boiled lobster and a baked, stuffed lobster served with drawn butter. You start off with the same lobster but change the end product substantially by adding high-fat ingredients in the preparation.

All seafood, prior to preparation, ranges from about 30–60 calories per cooked ounce. Cod, scallops, and monkfish are on the low calorie side whereas swordfish, salmon, and bluefish are on the higher calorie side due to their slightly higher fat content. Still, all are comparatively low in calories and fat compared to red meats. Even extra-lean ground beef usually rings in at about 75 calories per ounce cooked.

With the great emphasis today on lowering fat, saturated fat, and cholesterol intake, fish is a good choice. When comparing protein food choices, fin fish clearly comes out a winner in terms of percent of calories from fat and the low quantity of saturated fat. Unbeknownst to many, there is little difference in the quantity of dietary cholesterol between meats and seafood. Most fin fish and shellfish are relatively low in saturated fat and cholesterol. However, there are a few shellfish that, although still low in saturated fat, are higher in cholesterol than red meats.

The well-liked crustacean, shrimp, has taken a beating over the past several years as cholesterol consciousness has risen. Actually, shellfish in general have gotten a bad rap. Some of the beating is fair, but some is based on misconceptions. Shrimp is high in cholesterol, about 166 mg for a 3-ounce cooked portion. Compare that to red meat at about 72 mg of cholesterol for the same portion. As for other crustaceans and mollusks, squid (calamari) is even higher in cholesterol content than shrimp while clams, mussels, oysters, lobster, scallops, and crab are lower in cholesterol.

When considering the cholesterol content of shellfish, it is important to know that shellfish is quite low in saturated fat. It has about the same saturated fat content as fin fish. Also, when consumed in a low-fat recipe, shellfish is very low in calories. A major concept today holds that in eating for heart health, one should first reduce saturated fat intake as a way to lower blood cholesterol. So don't exclusively consider the cholesterol content of shellfish when contemplating menu choices. Remember that some shellfish is low in cholesterol, and all shellfish is low in saturated fat and calories. Think more about how that menu item is prepared; good choices are those using low fat preparation methods.

In addition to their health and calorie-counting benefits, in recent years it has been found that some fish, particularly the fattier ones, have a high quantity of fish oils. These fish oils are also called omega-3 fats. Fish that have a large quantity of omega-3 fats include salmon, bluefish, mackeral, sardines, rainbow trout, and eel (for those of you who consider eel a taste treat). There has been and continues to be much research on the omega-3 fats. They are categorized as polyunsaturated fats and have been found to have some beneficial effects on lowering triglyceride levels. The verdict is still out on the effects of omega-3 fats on blood cholesterol levels.

Fish has an additional health benefit in its low sodium content. Most fresh fin fish and shellfish are low in sodium compared to other protein foods: meat, cheese, and poultry. You'll find that a few items, such as surimi, crab, lobster, shrimp, mussels, and oysters, have slightly more sodium than other seafood. (Refer to the chart at the end of this chapter for nutrition information related to sodium.) Interestingly, there seems to be no correlation between the sodium content of salt water and fresh water seafood.

Obviously, the biggest problem with the sodium content of fish when dining out is the additional sodium that is added in preparation. Items such as soy sauce or tomato sauce can raise sodium dramatically. Also, the process of smoking can raise sodium content and bluefish, salmon, and mussels are frequently available smoked, often as appetizers.

Not only does fish offer a wide variety of tastes but it is also a healthy food for those with high blood pressure, heart disease, and weight problems as well as those simply striving for healthier eating habits. However, the healthy traits of seafood only remain so if low-fat cooking methods are used and accompaniments are in line with individual nutrition goals. Consider the low fat, low calorie, low cholesterol, and low sodium qualities of a seafood dinner consisting of poached salmon served with mustard dill sauce, baked potato, and salad with a tarragon vinaigrette dressing compared with the opposite extreme: a cup of fish chowder, a plate of fried clams, French fries, and creamy cole slaw. Obviously, just because it's seafood doesn't mean it's all great for you.

In fact, some of the fast food seafood shops offer some of the worst food choices available. Usually, the only choices are fried fish or fried shellfish. These items are served with French fries, fried onion rings, and/or creamy coleslaw. Until fast food fish chains decide to bake, broil, or boil some of their menu items, these stops are best passed by.

Think about exposing yourself to some new varieties of seafood, such as the increasingly popular mahi mahi (dolphin fish, no relation to the sea mammal),

monkfish, and mussels. So often people limit their seafood choices to the ones they grew up on—flounder,
cod, haddock, and shrimp. Many settle for the familiar frying or broiling with butter. Be adventurous and
try the many new and creative low-fat and low-calorie
preparation methods used today. Consider poached
salmon, steamed halibut and vegetables, barbecued
shrimp, mesquite grilled tuna, swordfish kabobs, and
blackened bluefish!

Managing the menu

You may have encountered menus listing blackened
bluefish, blackened redfish, blackened salmon, and
others. Blackening represents one of the hottest (literally) trends in seafood cookery to blossom over the last
few years—Cajun cuisine. Cajun cuisine includes both
creole cookery and blackening. These cooking techniques have taken restaurants by storm. There are
restaurants now that exclusively prepare Cajun cuisine, and there are many that simply have included
Cajun menu listings, such as shrimp creole and blackened fish, chicken, or beef. What's great is that both
creole cookery and blackened foods are healthy, and
best yet, loaded with pizazz.

Paul Prudhomme, the well known Cajun chef and
owner of K-Paul's restaurant in New Orleans, has
promoted these cooking techniques. Cajun cookery
has its roots with the French pioneers who originally
settled in Nova Scotia. These folks were driven out
of Canada by the British, and they finally settled in
the Louisiana bayou country, where Cajun cooking
traditions now continue.

Paul Prudhomme is best known for the blackening
technique. Blackening can be done to a variety of fin
fish and shellfish. The meatier fishes, such as swordfish and salmon, lend themselves better to blackening than the lighter, flaker species such as sole or
flounder. The cooking method uses only a small
amount of fat, which is placed in a very hot cast-iron
skillet prior to adding the fish. Hot spices, such as garlic powder, cayenne, and white pepper, are combined
to surround the exterior of the fish and form a bar-
rier between the food and hot skillet. The high heat
used for cooking evaporates the moisture, leaving the
outer fish fibers crusty with spice and the interior
juicy and flavorful.

Cajun cookery is great for adding lots of tasty spice while keeping calories low. Paul Prudhomme gave a true description of Cajun cuisine in a 1985 *Newsweek* article: "Cajun cooking is to stay just this side of the threshold between pleasure and pain. If you cross the threshold, people won't enjoy the food. If you stay this side of it, each bite leaves an aftertaste, and you want one more bite." Personally, my favorite is blackened salmon–the hotter, the better!

A relatively new kid on the block when it comes to seafood is surimi. This is the crabmeat look-alike that is substituted or used in combination with crabmeat for seafood salads and casseroles. Surimi is most often made out of pollack. From the seafood nutrition information chart at the end of the chapter, you can observe that surimi is low in calories, fat, and cholesterol but a bit higher in sodium than other fin fish. It also has a bit of sugar added in the manufacturing process, but not enough to cause concern for those who have diabetes. Surimi is much less expensive than crabmeat. If you spot a menu listing for "seafood" salad or sandwich instead of "crabmeat" salad or sandwich, be assured that a surimi product is being used alone or in combination with crabmeat or other shellfish.

Even though surimi starts off as a healthy food choice, it is often combined with mayonnaise in a seafood salad or with cream and/or cheese in a casserole; thus the calories skyrocket. So you may consider choosing surimi, but ask questions about its preparation prior to ordering and being surprised.

Another new trend in seafood restaurants is the "raw bar." Raw bars stock oysters, cherrystone or littleneck clams, which are usually served on the half shell, and the more exotic cerviche, sushi, or sashimi. Although they are referred to as raw bars, you will usually find many cooked, steamed, or marinated items such as shrimp, crab claws, clams, and mussels.

Before propping yourself up at the local raw bar, you should know about some cautions to be taken when eating raw fish. Due to the increased consumption of raw seafood in the United States over the last few years, there has been an increase in food-borne illnesses that have their origins in raw seafood. The infection resulting from eating tainted fin fish is anisakiasis. This results from a roundworm that lives in larvae form in the fish's organs. On rare occasion, the parasite makes its way into the flesh of the fish, and eventually to the raw bar. If the fish is cooked, the parasite is killed in the process. If served raw, obviously, it will not be killed prior to serving. There are other food-borne illnesses that can occur from eating raw shellfish. The home economists from the USDA meat and poultry hotline recommend completely avoiding all raw seafood. If you choose to consume raw seafood, practice caution. Make sure the restaurant does a large raw bar business and the fish appears very fresh, well refrigerated, and cleaned. Looks and smells tell it all.

For those monitoring their calories and saturated fat consumption, there are lots of good choices at the raw bar. Almost all items are appropriate. If they are served raw, obviously no fat has been used in preparation. Raw oysters, clams, sushi, and sashimi are served with very low-calorie sauces, such as seafood cocktail sauce, fresh lemon or lime, horseradish, or soy sauce (if monitoring sodium intake, be careful with the soy sauce). The cooked items may also be quite healthy and served in light sauces. Many are available marinated, barbecued, mesquite-grilled, or Cajun spiced. Try to avoid the drawn butter that often accompanies the steamed clams or mussels. Stick to using the next-to-no-calorie-broth that is also commonly served.

Consider ordering raw or healthfully cooked appetizers while your dining companions might be indulging in a high-fat, high-calorie bowl of New England clam chowder or fried calamari. Or think about having an appetizer as your main course. Order à la carte and have an appetizer, a baked potato or rice pilaf, and the house salad with dressing on the side to round out the meal.

As you sit with the menu in front of you, contemplating what you should have and what you want to have, remember to be a good fat detective. Look for the Green Flag Words that indicate lower fat and healthier preparation methods. Steer clear of the Red Flag Words that point out items or cooking styles with lots of fat and other unhealthy ingredients added.

Give consideration once again to the portion control strategy of sharing. One person might order a salad and appetizer or a shrimp salad plate and the other, a main course. By sharing both orders, you may better match your nutrition goals.

When the menu arrives, look for certain key words and phrases that signal the nutritional advisability of the items. We call them "Green Flag" (go for it) and "Red Flag" (steer clear) words.

Green Flag Words

broiled
blackened
Cajun style
in marinara sauce
sauteed in light wine sauce
mesquite-grilled; grilled
in spicy tomato sauce
in mustard dill sauce (ask if much
    mayonnaise is used)
with herbs, or spices, lemon, gar-
    lic, cilantro
marinated
barbecued
stir-fried (beware of increased
    sodium)
teriyaki (beware of increased
    sodium)
steamed
kabobs
served with gazpacho salsa

Red Flag Words

fried
deep-fried
breaded and fried
batter-dipped and fried
fish 'n chips
creamy; served in creamy wine
    sauce
served with cheese sauce
en casserole
lobster or seafood pie
Newburg
Thermidor
baked stuffed
stuffed and rolled
creamy chowder or bisque

**Special
Requests
Seafood
Style**

Please broil dry with a few bread crumbs.

Bring me a few extra lemon wedges.

Please serve the salad dressing on the side.

Do you have any interesting vinegars I could use on my salad?

Could I substitute a baked potato for French fries?

Could I substitute a dinner salad for the creamy cole slaw?

Please bring the butter and sour cream on the side.

Could I get a doggie bag at the beginning of my meal?

Please bring an extra plate; we are going to share.

Please bring my appetizer as my main course, but I'll have my salad with the others.

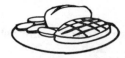

Typical Menu: Seafood Style

From the Raw Bar
- ✓**Oysters** on the halfshell served with fresh lemon and horseradish
- ✓**Cherrystone clams** on the half-shell served with cocktail sauce
- ✓**Assorted sashimi** served with wasabi, ginger root, and white rice
- ✓**Raw bar for two:** oysters, clams, crab claws, and shrimp

Appetizers
- **Baked clams Casino**
- ✓**Steamed clams** with broth and drawn butter
- **Cajun-fried calamari** served with spicy tomato sauce
- **Oysters rockefeller**
- ✓**Marinated calamari**
- ✓**Barbecued shrimp**
- **Scallops tempura**
- ✓**Shrimp cocktail**–6 large shrimp served with cocktail sauce

Soups
- ✓**Shrimp gumbo**
- **Fish chowder**
- **New England clam chowder**
- ✓**Manhattan clam chowder**
- **Lobster bisque**
- **Shrimp bisque**

Fin Fish Entrees*
The following fish are available prepared in several ways: broiled, steamed with vegetables, mesquite-grilled, blackened, or basted and grilled with teriyaki sauce:
- ✓**Bluefish**
- ✓**Haddock**
- ✓**Halibut**

✓*Preferred Choice*

✓**Mahi mahi** (dolphin fish)
✓**Monkfish**
✓**Redfish**
✓**Salmon**
✓**Swordfish**
The following fish are available prepared fried or Cajun-fried:
Bass
Catfish
Flounder
Haddock
✓**Broiled mackeral** with light mustard and dill sauce
Baked stuffed gray or lemon sole
Scrod, stuffed and baked, served in cheese sauce
✓**Swordfish kabobs** (choice of one or two kabobs, with marinated swordfish pieces, skewered with peppers, mushrooms, and red onions)

Shellfish Entrees*

Baked stuffed jumbo shrimp
Seafood casserole (crabmeat, shrimp, scallops, and others combined with Parmesan cheese cream sauce and topped with breadcrumbs)
✓**Boiled Maine lobster** with drawn butter and lemon, served complete with corn on the cob, creamy coleslaw, and watermelon for dessert
Lobster pie (lobster meat combined in cream sauce and served in a casserole topped with breadcrumbs)
✓**Scallops** sauteed in spicy tomato sauce
✓**Alaskan king crab** claws steamed and served with drawn butter

✓**Cioppino** (clams, shrimp, lobster,
and calamari braised in tomato
sauce and served over pasta)
✓**Bouillabaisse** (seafood stew with
monkfish, cod, and lobster)

*Note: All entrees are served
with a choice of two of the following items:

French fries
✓**Baked potato**
✓**Saffron rice**
✓**Rice pilaf**
✓**Tossed green salad**
Creamy coleslaw
✓**Sauteed zucchini,** yellow squash,
and onion
✓**Steamed fresh broccoli** with
lemon wedges

Desserts **Creamy New York cheesecake**
✓**Fresh strawberries** or raspber-
ries served with crème de casis
and whipped cream
✓**Watermelon**
Chocolate layer cake
Apple pie à la mode with
vanilla ice cream

Now that you've seen what may be available on the
menu, look over the following five "Model Meals" for
suggestions on how to order to achieve specific nutritional goals. Models are numbered one to five for
quick reference and each is followed by an "Estimated
Nutrient Evaluation" that analyzes the content of
that meal.

May I Take Your Order

Healthy	30% Calories as fat
Daily	20% Calories as protein
Eating	50% Calories as carbohydrate
Goals	300 mg/day Cholesterol
	3000 mg/day Sodium

❶
Low Calorie/	**Tossed green salad** (hold dress-
Low Fat	ing; request lemon wedges)
Model Meal	*Quantity:* 2 cups
	Exchanges: 2 vegetables
	Swordfish kabobs
	Quantity: 1 skewer
	Exchanges: 4 meat (lean); 1 fat; 1
	vegetable
	Rice pilaf
	Quantity: 1 cup
	Exchanges: 3 starch; 1 fat
	Coffee or tea
	Quantity: 1 cup
	Exchanges: free

Estimated	530 calories
Nutrient	23% calories as fat
Evaluation	32% calories as protein
	45% calories as carbohydrate
	70 mg cholesterol
	670 mg sodium

Low Calorie/ Low Cholesterol Model Meal

Tossed green salad
Quantity: 2 cups
Vinaigrette, lemon-basil (on the side)
Quantity: 1 tbsp
Sauteed scallops in spicy tomato sauce
Quantity: 1½ cups
Saffron rice
Quantity: ⅔ cup
Broccoli, steamed fresh (hold butter)
Quantity: ½ cup

Estimated Nutrient Evaluation

540 calories
31% calories as fat
31% calories as protein
38% calories as carbohydrate
60 mg cholesterol
1100 mg sodium

Higher Calorie/Low Fat Model Meal

Barbecued shrimp on skewer (10)
Quantity: ½ order
Exchanges: 2 meat (lean)
Hard roll with butter
Quantity: 1 roll; 1 pat
Exchanges: 1 starch; 1 fat
Blackened redfish
Quantity: 4 oz
Exchanges: 4 meat (lean)
Baked potato with sour cream
Quantity: 1 potato; 2 tbsp sour cream
Exchanges: 3 starch; 1 fat
Sauteed zucchini, yellow squash, and onions
Quantity: 1 cup
Exchanges: 1 fat; 2 vegetables

Fresh raspberries with crème de
casis (hold whipped cream)
Quantity: 1 cup
Exchanges: 2 fruit

Estimated   836 calories
Nutrient   22% calories as fat
Evaluation   28% calories as protein
                50% calories as carbohydrate
                190 mg cholesterol
                1200 mg sodium

---

❹
Higher   **New England Clam Bake:**
Calorie/Low   **Fish chowder**
Cholesterol   *Quantity:* ½ cup
Model Meal   **Steamed clams** and drawn butter
                with lemon and clam broth
                Quantity: 10–15 clams; 2 tsp sauce
                Boiled Maine lobster with
                drawn butter and lemon
                Quantity: 1¼-lb. lobster; 2 tsp
                sauce
                Corn on the cob (hold butter and
                salt)
                Quantity: 2 ears
                Creamy coleslaw
                Quantity: 1 cup
                Watermelon
                Quantity: 2 cups

Estimated   850 calories
Nutrient   31% calories as fat
Evaluation   29% calories as protein
                41% calories as carbohydrate
                165 mg cholesterol
                1350 mg sodium

❺

Low Sodium Model Meal

Shrimp with cocktail sauce
Quantity: 3 large shrimp; 2 tbsp sauce
Hard roll
Quantity: 1
Salmon, mesquite-grilled with Cajun vegetables
Quantity: 4 oz salmon; 1 cup vegetables
Baked potato with butter
Quantity: 1 potato; 1 tsp butter
Lemon herbal tea
Quantity: 2 cups

Estimated Nutrient Evaluation

727 calories
33% calories as fat
28% calories as protein
39% calories as carbohydrate
160 mg cholesterol
950 mg sodium

Nutrition Information about Selected Seafoods +

Food Item	Por- tion (ozs)*	Total Cals.	% Cals. As Fat	% Sat. Fat	% Poly- unsat. Fat	% Mono- unsat. Fat	Cholest- erol (mg)	Sodi- um (mg)
Fin Fish								
bass	3	129	29	21	29	38	77	79
bluefish	3	140	31	21	25	42	66	68
catfish	3	132	32	23	24	38	65	72
cod (scrod)	3	93	7	19	34	14	49	61
flounder/ sole	3	104	12	24	28	20	55	92
haddock	3	98	7	16	33	16	65	77
halibut	3	119	19	14	32	33	35	59
mackeral	3	232	60	23	34	29	80	101
mahi mahi (dolphin fish)	3	97	7	26	23	16	83	99
monkfish	3	85	17	n/a	n/a	n/a	28	21
perch (redfish)	3	103	16	14	26	37	46	82

Nutrition Information about Selected Seafoods+
(Continued)

Food Item	Por- tion (ozs)*	Total Cals.	% Cals. As Fat	% Sat. Fat	% Poly- unsat. Fat	% Mono- unsat. Fat	Cholest- erol (mg)	Sodi- um (mg)
Fin Fish (Continued)								
pompano	3	179	52	37	12	27	54	65
salmon (sockeye)	3	183	45	17	23	48	74	56
surimi (crab- like)	3	84	8	n/a	n/a	n/a	25	122
swordfish	3	132	30	27	23	38	43	98
trout (rainbow)	3	129	25	19	35	30	62	29
tuna (fresh)	3	123	8	25	30	16	51	41
Shellfish								
Crustaceans								
crab (Alaskan)	3	82	15	9	35	12	45	911
lobster	3	83	5	18	14	26	61	323
shrimp	3	84	10	26	40	15	166	190
Mollusks								
clams	3	126	12	10	28	48	57	95
mussels	3	147	23	18	27	23	48	313
oysters	3	117	32	25	30	10	93	190
scallops	3	100	8	11	5	34	37	182
squid	3	104	14	25	37	8	264	49
For Reference								
beef, round (lean example)	3	181	38	46	5	49	72	51
prime rib (high fat example)	3	328	77	47	4	49	72	51

+Information obtained from "Composition of Foods,"
United States Department of Agriculture, Human Nutrition Information Services. Agricultural Handbook Sources,
8-15 "Finfish and Shellfish," 8-13 "Beef Products."
*3 ounces cooked is estimated to be about 4 ounces of raw
quantity.

7

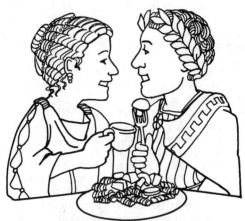

Healthier eating out
Italian Style
with special PIZZA section

For many Americans, Italian cuisine is on their best-seller list when it comes to dining out. Whether it be parmigiana, cacciatore, scampi, primavera, or piccata, there's a wonderful world of taste treats at Italian restaurants. And many items, in fact, are very healthy. Italian food, according to the National Restaurant Association, is one of our most popular ethnic cuisines. Over the years, Italian dishes have become woven into American culture. Today, foods thought of as Italian in origin are considered standard in many American family-style restaurants. For instance, the restaurant chain TGI Friday's lists pizza and chicken parmigiana on their regular menu.

Italian food is eaten in a wide price range of restaurants from cheap eats to elegant dining. Pizza is one of the most commonly eaten Italian foods, and it's often enjoyed quite inexpensively (see separate section on pizza below). There are several nationwide chains specializing in inexpensive Italian food: Papa Gino's and Pizza Hut are two examples. In most cities and towns you'll find at least one small, family-run Italian restaurant offering great home-cooked pasta, tomato sauces, meatballs, hard-crusted Italian bread, and carafes of Chianti—all served on the traditional red-and-white-checkered tablecloth. Some cities have a certain section where Italian restaurants, groceries, and after-dinner espresso and dessert spots abound, such as Little Italy in New York City and the North End in Boston.

On the upscale side, there are certainly many expensive and elegant Italian restaurants spread around the country. They often specialize in food from particular regions of Italy and integrate some of the newer ingredients and cooking methods into their menus. I call them "nouvelle Italian." Some of these cooking methods, such as grilling or adding sun-dried tomatoes, are actually more American than Italian. But it all gets interwoven into what we think of as Italian food.

Interestingly, the difference between what Americans and Italians regard as Italian food may be tremendous, especially among traditional Italian chefs. There are differences in the types of foods eaten, when meals are eaten, and even in the order in which foods are served. Over the years, Italian food in America has certainly been influenced by American taste buds and our style of eating. In fact, when many Americans think of Italian food, they conjure up images of spaghetti with tomato sauce and meatballs or **veal parmigiana**. In actuality, those dishes are examples of Southern Italian cooking. Some people even say that meatballs are an American invention and not an Italian tradition at all.

In learning about Italian food, you soon realize that there are broad distinctions between Northern and Southern style Italian cooking. Over the years, Southern cuisine has been more familiar to Americans. Tomato sauces—marinara and cacciatore—are commonly used along with olive oil, oregano, and garlic. Northern Italian cuisine is becoming more well known in America today, and it is often seen in up-scale Italian restaurants. In the broad picture, Northern cuisine is lighter and makes use of wine sauces, light cream, and butter sauces; marsala and scampi are representative of Northern cooking. Both Northern and Southern style cooking have their healthy and not-so-healthy aspects.

Many Italians and Italian chefs chuckle at this American distinction between Southern and Northern Italian cooking. In reality, Italian cooking styles, ingredients, and dishes have their origins in many different regions of Italy. Polenta, for instance, came from the Po Valley, and heavy use of spinach and olive oil is typical of the Tuscany region. When the roots of Italian cooking are examined, one realizes that the origins of cooking styles are directly related to ingredients produced in that area.

As society grows increasingly more mobile, cooking styles, like people, migrate from one region to another. As chefs from America travel around Italy tasting different regional cuisines, they bring many dishes back and integrate them into new menu selections. Of late, our American view of Italian food has broadened. Just one example is the use of a much wider variety of pastas. Tortellini, fusilli, cannelloni, and angel hair are showing up more frequently on restaurant menus. Beyond the many different sizes and shapes of pasta, you now also find tomato, spinach, sage, and whole-wheat pasta to choose among. (See the "Know Your Pasta" section at the end of this chapter.)

Beyond the differences between what Americans and Italians think of as Italian food, there are big differences in eating styles. Traditionally in Italy, and still often today, the big meal of the day was consumed in the afternoon. Historically, shops and businesses close about midday, and people take time to enjoy their afternoon meal. The meal is begun with an antipasto, which simply means "before the meal." The first course, referred to as *primo piatto,* often consists of either a pasta dish or soup, perhaps a minestrone. The *secondo piatto,* or second course, consists of meat, fish, or poultry and is often served with one vegetable. Bread is also served at this point. Unlike American protocol, the salad, or *insalata,* is served after the second course.

An Italian chef in a local restaurant told me that it would be hard to serve a salad *after* the meal to Americans. It is not a familiar custom here, and he jokingly said that most customers are too anxious to eat and would not wait 15 to 20 minutes for their first course if they did not receive a salad. In Italy, after the salad course is eaten, a fruit or cheese platter is served. There is really little attention to sweet desserts in Italy within the context of the meal. But certainly Italy is well known for its *gelati*!

What to consider before ordering

As always, the choice is yours whether to eat a healthy meal and come out of the restaurant feeling pleasantly sated or to go for broke (and fat) and come out with that post-Thanksgiving stuffed-turkey feeling. Italian meals, eaten in a variety of Italian restaurants from inexpensive to costly, can range from healthy to nutritional disaster. Consider the following healthy Italian meal: a cup of minestrone or stracciatelle; linguine with white clam sauce; and, as enjoyed in Italy, a demitasse of espresso. At the opposite end of the spectrum, consider this high fat, cholesterol, and sodium meal: several pieces of Italian garlic bread doused in olive oil; an antipasto of various Italian cheeses, Genoa salami, marinated artichokes, and olives; an entree of fettucini Alfredo; and the well-known Italian dessert, cannoli. Obviously, you have a wide range of choices.

The challenges for dining healthy on Italian food are obvious. But with a bit of knowledge, putting some skills into action, and practicing some behavioral strategies, you can continue to enjoy your Italian favorites and possibly even experience some new taste sensations. This is true whether you are watching cholesterol, fat, sodium, sugar, or calories—singly or together.

The strategy of sharing in an Italian restaurant can be quite helpful. If you have a willing dining companion, sharing allows you to taste and enjoy several items while minimizing the portions you consume. In fact, a friend and I recently ate in the Italian restaurant Filomena in Washington, DC. We practiced the art of sharing and portion control by each ordering an insalata tricolore, which consisted of green arugula, white endive, and red radicchio, followed by an entree of linguine with bacon, onion, basil, and tomatoes. We then split a decadent chocolate dessert. We each had a cup of coffee and a sip of Amaretto to complete the meal . . . *Delizioso!*

Think about sharing straight through the meal. Start with an antipasto, such as mussels marinara, or split a salad, perhaps of marinated seafood. Think about sharing a pasta dish, or have one person order a pasta dish while the other orders a seafood or poultry dish. If you can afford the calories and it's appropriate to your specific dietary modifications, split a dessert, maybe even four ways. After all, a taste is usually all you really want.

Managing the menu

As the menu is placed before you, the great, crusty Italian bread and a crock of creamy butter also appear. If you find that the first piece of bread and butter simply gets you started on a downhill course, try to avoid it altogether. If your calories and meal plan allow, consider having one piece of bread with minimal or no butter. Then make sure the bread and butter are passed away from you and remain at the other end of the table. Practice the out-of-sight, out-of-mind theory. Another option, if your dining partners are willing, is to have the bread and butter simply removed from the table. Again, don't be afraid to be a trend setter—most people will thank you. As you probably realize, the garlic bread dripping with olive oil is best to avoid entirely. It is addictive and quite high in calories due to the high fat content of the oil.

If calories should be kept on the low side, you are probably best off simply focusing on an appropriate entree and a fresh green salad. If you have more calories and fat to "spend," you might consider an antipasto or soup. There usually is a broad variety of antipasto choices from healthy to disastrous. Among the healthy options, consider squid, mussels, or clams in a lemon-garlic-herb-wine-butter (any combination) sauce. Or maybe they are available in a marinara concoction, which is a light tomato sauce. There might even be an antipasto simply consisting of marinated vegetables. Avoid the deep-fried mozzarella sticks, meats, and cheeses and heavy cream sauces.

On occasion, you might consider ordering an antipasto or appetizer-size serving of pasta as your entree. Sometimes, in more authentically Italian restaurants, the pasta is listed separately, and the portions are appetizer-size because it is thought that you will order a primo piatto of pasta and a secondo piatto of meat or seafood. Some menus will say "These are entree portions; appetizer portions are also available." Or if the menu states "Every pasta is available as a dinner for an additional charge," you will know that the listings are appetizer-size servings. That's perfect for assisting you in limiting your portion. Simply choose to have a cup of soup or a salad while others might be consuming their antipasto or pasta; then have your antipasto or appetizer-size pasta when they are eating their secondo piatto.

Insalata, the innocent sounding, good, crunchy greens, are filling and low calorie—maybe, depending on the listings of each Italian menu. There often are many salads to choose among. Look for those made with radicchio, arugula, endive, tomatoes, broccoli, mixed greens, spinach, beets, peppers, onions, and other raw vegetables. A few olives or the nouvelle items—sun-dried tomatoes or pignoli (pine) nuts—will not present much of a problem. However, there are high-fat ingredients lurking in many Italian salads. Watch out for the Caesar salad with egg, grated cheese, anchovies, and oily dressing. Other high-fat, high-cholesterol items might be cheeses, pasta, ham, bacon, and nuts. Order dressing on the side, and look for a light dressing such as a vinaigrette; better yet, try a bit of olive oil with vinegar or fresh lemon wedges. Some of the more contemporary Italian restaurants are using new, interesting vinegars such as balsamic, tarragon, and lemon-basil. If you spot it on the menu, perhaps used in some dish, it is likely that you can order some on the side to sprinkle on your salad.

Moving on to the main course, try to choose either a pasta dish or a meat, seafood, or poultry selection. (Remember the idea of splitting entrees with your dining companion.) Pasta is made from combining flour, water, and (optionally) eggs. So there is a minimal amount of cholesterol and fat (from the egg yolk) in pasta. Pasta is made into many different shapes and forms, some large, some small, some stuffed, some not. (See "Know Your Pasta" at the end of this chapter.)

Generally speaking, there has been a good deal of negative press about pasta over the years related to its fattening qualities. The reality is that pasta, it-self, has almost no fat. It is basically carbohydrate with a bit of protein. The problems occur when pasta gets topped or stuffed with high-fat ingredients— cheeses, sausage, creams, bacon, etc. So the challenge in choosing a pasta dish is to keep an eye out for the "go-ahead-and-order" words: herbs, spices, garlic, wine sauce, light tomato sauce, etc. (See Green Flag Words below.)

There are a great many healthy pasta choices. Look for marinara, primavera (sauteed vegetables), red or white clam sauces, calamari sauce, mushrooms and wine sauce, tomato and basil. Try to avoid the stuffed pastas such as tortellini, ravioli, cannelloni, manicotti, agnolotti, and lasagne. These are often stuffed with high-fat ingredients. Served under a light sauce, you're best off with angel hair, linguine, fusilli, fettucini, or ziti. Try some of the interestingly flavored green, red, or whole-wheat pastas that are being used with increasing frequency. These might provide a new, healthy taste treat.

For people carefully counting calories and fat, pesto sauces should be avoided. Pesto is typically made with basil (that's a good start), but then pignolo (pine) nuts, olive oil, and lots of Parmesan cheese are added. Just because it's green doesn't mean it's low in calories. If you've got a few calories to spare and you eat a limited quantity, pesto sauce is a possibility, however.

One of the newer Italian taste treats to make its way onto many menus is risotto. Risotto is a creamy, short-grain rice with stubby kernels. It traces its ancestry to the Po Valley region of Italy where it is grown in abundance. Unfortunately, it is often prepared with lots of butter and cheese, so the taste is great but the fat, calories, and cholesterol might be high. If you wish to try it, look for risotto that has been prepared with spices and vegetables.

Polenta is another new item being served in some upscale Italian restaurants. It is almost like a corn meal pudding, made simply from corn meal, water, and salt. Polenta is a staple in the Veneto region of Italy. It is typically served with sauces, many of which, unfortunately, contain high-fat ingredients, for instance, sausage or herring.

Whether it is *pollo, pesce,* or *carne,* that is, poultry, seafood, or meat, there are many good entree choices. In general, if you are closely watching your cholesterol and saturated fat intake, you should choose among fish, scallops, and chicken. You are also well advised to stay with these choices if calories are your bottom line. Again, as with pasta, the magic words to look for are tomato sauces, mushroom or wine sauces, lemon and butter sauce, seasoned with garlic and herbs, cacciattore, scampi, and marsala.

When choosing your entree, you'll want to avoid the high-fat and high-sodium prosciutto ham, pancetta (Italian cured bacon), various cheeses, and cream sauces. Shrimp is fine to order on occasion. There are usually some nice low-calorie and low-fat shrimp dishes on every Italian menu. Shrimp are high in cholesterol, but they are fine if eaten infrequently. Interestingly, calamari (squid) is also high in cholesterol content. (For further nutrient information on seafood, see Chapter 6.)

If you are offered a side dish of pasta with your entree, you may be asked to choose between a marinara sauce or garlic oil. From a calorie and fat standpoint, you are better off with the marinara sauce. Also consider having nothing put on the pasta, and think about mixing it with the sauce from your entree.

A popular entree to order in an Italian restaurant is veal. There are some misconceptions about veal. Many people think veal is relatively low in calories, fat, and cholesterol. It is true that veal cutlet, often the very lean cut of veal used in Italian cooking, is low in calories (about 40–50 per oz), but the cholesterol content is similar to lean beef (about 20–25 mg/oz cooked). The other problem when ordering veal is that it's prepared most often by being dredged in flour and then sauteed. If you have a few extra calories to spare, veal marsala, cacciatore, or piccata might be a good choice. But if calories are tight, veal should be avoided and enjoyed at home where you can prepare it with minimal fat.

The commonly used oil in Italian cooking is olive oil. This is rooted in the prevalance of olives in Italy. Olives have been and still are plentiful. The use of olives and olive oil is therefore interwoven into many recipes. Recently, olive oil has received a lot of media attention. This is due to the fact that it is mainly a monounsaturated fat. Monounsaturated fats are now thought to help lower blood cholesterol; therefore, you are encouraged to use more of these oils. In addition, because olive oil is not an animal-based oil, it does not contain any cholesterol. So, in general, it is a healthy choice when selecting one oil over another. However, olive oil contains the same number of calories as every other oil and is 100 percent fat. So if calories and fat are your concern, you are still better off trying to eliminate as much olive oil, or any oil, as possible.

The end to many meals in America is a sweet dessert; that is not true in Italy. But because Italians have bent toward American ways when it comes to dessert, menus often contain items such as spumoni, cannoli, tortoni, and Italian ices to whet your taste buds. If your meal plan allows, you might want to think about splitting a dessert, or else choose the lower calorie and low-fat Italian ices or a fruit-based dessert. Another option is simply to end the meal as they do in Italy, with a demitasse of espresso, or, as in America, with a cup of coffee. If you have a few calories to spare and a liqueur fits into your dietary modifications, you might want to request a jigger (1½ oz) of Amaretto or Kahlua for your coffee (about 150 calories; no fat or cholesterol and negligible sodium). This might provide the finishing touch you're craving without the calories and fat of a decadent chocolate dessert. (See Chapter 19 for more information on drinks.)

When the menu arrives, look for certain key words and phrases that signal the nutritional advisability of the items. We call them "Green Flag" (go for it) and "Red Flag" (steer clear) words.

Green Flag Words

lightly sauteed with onions
shallots
peppers and mushrooms
artichoke hearts
sun-dried tomatoes
spicy marinara sauce
tomato-based sauce—marinara or cacciatore
light red sauce
light red-or-white-wine sauce
light mushroom sauce
capers

herbs and spices
garlic and oregano crushed toma-
    toes and spices
florentine (spinach)
grilled (often done to fish)
red or white clam sauce
primavera (make sure there is no
    cream sauce)
lemon sauce
piccata

**Red Flag
Words**

Alfredo
carbonara
saltimbocca
parmigiana
pancetta
oil
stuffed with cheese
stuffed with ricotta cheese
prosciutto
mozzarella cheese
percorino cheese (Romano)
creamy wine sauce
creamy cheese or mushroom sauce
made with three varieties of
    cheese
egg and cheese batter
fried
veal sausage
manicotti
cannelloni
lasagne
ravioli

**Special
Requests
Italian
Style**

Please don't put the bread down here.

Please remove my plate, I'm finished now.

I'll take the rest of this home in a doggie bag.

Would you ask the chef to remove the skin from the chicken.

Please hold the Parmesan cheese (or grated cheese), bacon, olives, pine nuts.

Hold the sauce on the pasta.

Please use only a small amount of sauce over the pasta.

Please serve the salad dressing on the side.

I'd like the appetizer-size pasta, and please bring that when you bring the other entrees.

Would you ask the chef to avoid using any extra salt.

PIZZA

How can you talk about Italian food without mentioning the most popular dish of all—Pizza! Pizza is almost as American as apple pie. There probably isn't a town or city in the United States where you can't at least get a cheese and tomato pizza. Pizza is eaten for lunch, for dinner, and (as I recall from college days) for quite a few late night snacks. Some people even eat leftover pizza for breakfast. Actually, not a bad nutritional choice.

Pizza can be part of a quick and relatively inexpensive meal out, or it can be picked up for a speedy meal on the homefront. Pizza is historically one of the most commonly home-delivered foods. Lots of pizza is purchased at local pizza parlors, where you'll also discover a long list of submarine sandwiches, which are discussed in Chapter 16. At pizza parlors you can take your choice from a wide array of toppings, including the common onion, mushrooms, sausage, and pepperoni items. Pizza is also the mainstay of several fast food chains, such as Papa Gino's and Pizza Hut. Today, pizza is even well integrated into the menus of American family-style restaurants.

There are restaurants today specializing in certain types of pizzas, such as deep dish, often referred to as Chicago pizza or stuffed pizza. Pizzeria Uno, with many locations around the country, specializes in what they call "Chicago's original deep-dish pizza." There is a chain of pizza restaurants in Massachusetts called Bertucci's, which uses brick ovens to bake their pizzas over an open flame.

There seems to be a move afoot to be more creative with ingredients and the combinations of items used on pizza. That's great for the nutrition conscious because many of the new ingredients are vegetables and other lower-calorie items (see Green Flag Pizza Toppings). The great spicy taste of pizza can be retained while reducing the fat, cholesterol, sodium, and calories contained in extra cheese, sausage, and pepperoni.

From a nutritional standpoint, pizza is often thought of as off-limits. People contemplating weight loss and eventual maintenance think there is no pizza in their future, ever! That is simply not true. The biggest nutritional problem with pizza is that it's easy to eat too much. There is usually another piece waiting in front of you, and it's hard to resist just one more slice.

Think about it. Pizza dough is basically flour, yeast, salt, and water—no fat, no cholesterol, few calories. Then a tomato sauce is added—another low-calorie item. Next, the cheese is spread, which, of course, is high in calories and fat. But how much cheese is really on one slice of pizza—¾ to 1 ounce? The final step is to add other toppings. Will they be low-calorie mushrooms, onions, spinach, and tomato slices, or will you order extra cheese, pepperoni, and anchovies? Knowing more about the nutritional content of pizza, it is interesting to observe how a "weight watcher" eats pizza. Typically, they will avoid the crust and eat the high-fat, high-cholesterol contents. They'd be better off doing the reverse for both the calorie and health reasons.

The point to be made is that pizza need not be a nutritional disaster. Initially, you simply have to think about what extras you'll add. It's best to set a limit of two to four extra items. Then you must decide how many pieces are appropriate for you to eat within the context of your nutritional goals. Obviously, if you are attempting to lose weight, one or two slices might be plenty. If cholesterol is your concern and you choose ingredients wisely, perhaps three or four slices will be no problem. It is also helpful not to order a bigger-size pizza than is needed. There will be extra pieces staring you in the face, and that just promotes overeating.

Another bit of advice: have a salad along with the pizza. A salad will help you fill up on lower calorie, healthy greens, and it won't leave as much room for pizza. Most restaurants serving pizza also have salads; even corner pizza parlors offer at least a garden or Greek salad. Crunch on the salad first, prior to diving into the pizza. Pizzeria Uno offers their Ike's house salad, which is a nice light salad with mushrooms, tomatoes, and rings of onion and pepper. It's also served with Ike's dressing on the side, a light oil-and-vinegar mixture. One of my clients intent on maintaining a 50-pound weight loss, recounted her Pizzeria Uno pizza dinner in a weight maintenance group: "I had a large green salad, with dressing that is always served on the side, and two pieces of deep-dish pizza with broccoli, onions, and feta cheese. Of course, I could have eaten more, but I felt pleasantly sated."

There are really many tasty, low-fat and low-calorie toppings with which to load your pizza. Choose among healthy ingredients such as spinach, mushrooms, broccoli, and roasted peppers, simply to name a few. Most of the ingredients on the Red Flag Pizza Toppings list should be avoided due to their calorie, sodium, fat, and cholesterol content. Items such as ham or hamburger are better meat choices for those whose main concerns are not calories. There are many other pizza toppings that, although a bit higher in calories, fat, and sodium, are fine to use. These include black olives, feta cheese, and eggplant (which is often fried prior to being placed on the pizza), plus all of the "Green Flags" below.

Green Flag Pizza Toppings

green peppers
red peppers
roasted peppers
onions
sliced tomatoes
mushrooms
black olives
broccoli
eggplant
pineapple
tuna
garlic
feta cheese
spinach
chicken
shrimp or crabmeat
artichoke hearts

Red Flag Pizza Toppings

extra cheese
pepperoni
sausage
anchovies
bacon
meatballs
prosciutto
mozzarella cheese

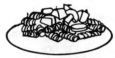

Typical Menu: Italian Style

Antipasto   **Antipasto for Two**–a combina-
tion of marinated mushrooms, ar-
tichoke hearts, Genoa salami, and
percorino cheese
Prosciutto wrapped around
melon
✓**Marinated calamari**
Garlic bread
✓**Marinated mushrooms**
Fried calamari
✓**Clams** steamed in white wine
Fried mozzarella sticks with
marinara sauce

Zuppa   ✓**Tortellini in broth**
✓**Pasta e fagioli** (bean and pasta
soup)
✓**Minestrone**
Lentil and sausage

Insalata   ✓**Arugula and Belgian endive**
served with balsamic vinaigrette
dressing
✓**Insalata frutte di mare** (marinated seafood, scallops, shrimp,
and calamari in a light marinade,
served on a bed of greens)
✓**Insalata di casa** (house salad
with greens, tomato, and onion)
Caesar salad (greens with but-
tery croutons, Parmesan cheese,
and a creamy Caesar dressing)

✓*Preferred Choice*

Pasta   **Cannelloni** stuffed with ricotta
cheese and spinach, topped with a
light tomato sauce
✓**Ziti Bolognese** (tubular noodles
topped with a light tomato sauce
of sauteed meat, celery, carrots,
and onions)
Fettucini Alfredo (thin, flat
pasta served with a creamy
cheese sauce)
✓**Angel hair** with white clam
sauce (the thinnest and lightest
pasta, served with a white-wine-
based sauce containing whole
clams)
Linguine with Gorgonzola (flat,
thin pasta served with a creamy
Gorgonzola cheese sauce)
✓**Fusilli primavera** (a spiral, long
pasta topped with a blend of spicy
sauteed seasonal vegetables)

Carne*   **Veal piccata** (medallions of veal
lightly sauteed in a butter, lemon,
and wine sauce)
✓**Veal cacciatore** (veal cutlet
topped with tomato sauce and
sauteed onions, mushrooms, and
peppers)
✓**Chicken primavera** (breast of
chicken lightly sauteed and
topped with sauteed seasonal
vegetables)
Veal saltimbocca (medallions of
veal filled with prosciutto ham,
sage, and mushrooms and topped
with mozzarella cheese)
Chicken parmigiana (chicken
cutlet baked with mozzarella
cheese and tomato sauce)
✓**Chicken in wine sauce** (sauteed
breast of chicken, roasted peppers,
and mushrooms, with Burgundy
wine, fresh garlic, and rosemary)

Pesce*   ✓**Shrimp primavera** (sauteed
shrimp and garden vegetables
served on top of a bed of angel
hair pasta)

✓**Shrimp marinara** (shrimp lightly
sauteed in garlic and topped with
tomato sauce)

Lobster in mushroom sauce (a
creamy porcini mushroom sauce
with large chunks of lobster tail)

Scallops marsala (sauteed scallops in a mushroom and marsala
wine sauce)

Shrimp scampi (shrimp sauteed
in olive oil, fresh garlic, white
wine, lemon, and oregano)

✓**Sole primavera** (fillet of sole sauteed with an assortment of seasonal fresh vegetables, zucchini,
peppers, and tomatoes)

*Above items served with a bowl of spaghetti
topped with your choice of marinara sauce or
olive oil and garlic.

Dolce   **Spumoni**
Cannoli
✓**Italian ice**
Tortoni

Now that you've seen what may be available on the
menu, look over the following five "Model Meals" for
suggestions on how to order to achieve specific nutritional goals. Models are numbered one to five for
quick reference, and each is followed by an "Estimated
Nutrient Evaluation" that analyzes the content of
that meal.

May I Take Your Order

Healthy	30% Calories as fat
Daily	20% Calories as protein
Eating	50% Calories as carbohydrate
Goals	300 mg/day Cholesterol
	3000 mg/day Sodium

❶

Low Calorie/	**Arugula and Belgian endive**
Low Fat	salad (request balsamic vinegar
Model Meal	on the side)
	Quantity: 2 cups
	Exchanges: 2 vegetable
	Fusilli (hold sauce and use that
	from entree)
	Quantity: 1 cup
	Exchanges: 2 starch
	Shrimp primavera (eat half)
	Quantity: 1½ cups
	Exchanges: 3–4 meat (lean); 2 fat;
	2 vegetable
	Espresso
	Quantity: 1 cup
	Exchanges: free

Estimated	450 calories
Nutrient	21% calories as fat
Evaluation	34% calories as protein
	45% calories as carbohydrate
	160 mg cholesterol
	650 mg sodium

❷
Low Calorie/ Low Cholesterol Model Meal

Marinated mushrooms
Quantity: 1 cup
Ziti Bolognese
Quantity: 1½ cups
Parmesan cheese for above
Quantity: 1 tbsp
Coffee
Quantity: 1 cup or more

Estimated Nutrient Evaluation

550 calories
32% calories as fat
20% calories as protein
47% calories as carbohydrate
55 mg cholesterol
1100 mg sodium

❸
Higher Calorie/Low Fat Model Meal

Special-request salad with red leaf lettuce, green peppers, mushrooms, tomatoes, black olives, onion, sprinkle of mozzarella
Quantity: 2 cups
Exchanges: 2 vegetable
Olive oil and vinegar dressing (on the side)
Quantity: 1 tsp oil; 2 tbsp vinegar
Exchanges: 1 fat (from the oil)
Pizza topped with sauteed chicken strips, roasted peppers, onions, white wine, oregano, feta cheese
Quantity: 2 slices
Exchanges: 3 meat; 2 fat; 2 vegetable; 4 starch

Estimated Nutrient Evaluation	780 calories
	36% calories as fat
	22% calories as protein
	42% calories as carbohydrate
	95 mg cholesterol
	1170 mg sodium

❹

Higher Calorie/Low Cholesterol Model Meal	**Tortellini in broth**
	Quantity: 1 cup
	Insalata di casa (dressing on the side)
	Quantity: 1 cup
	Basil vinaigrette dressing (on the side)
	Quantity: 1 tbsp
	Veal cacciatore
	Quantity: ½ portion (½ in doggie bag)
	Spaghetti (hold sauce and use that from entree)
	Quantity: 1½ cups
	Coffee with Kahlua (hold whipped cream)
	Quantity: 1 cup

Estimated Nutrient Evaluation	870 calories
	29% calories as fat
	22% calories as protein
	41% calories as carbohydrate
	8% calories as alcohol
	100 mg cholesterol
	1050 mg sodium

❺

Low Sodium Model Meal	**Clams** steamed in white wine
	Quantity: 10 clams (½ order)
	Linguini with Gorgonzola (hold sauce and use that from entree)
	Quantity: 1½ cups

Chicken in wine sauce (request limited additional salt)
Quantity: ½ portion (½ in doggie bag)
Italian ice
Quantity: 1 cup

Estimated Nutrient Evaluation	
	810 calories
	32% calories as fat
	15% calories as protein
	53% calories as carbohydrate
	170 mg cholesterol
	680 mg sodium

Know your pastas

Pasta, meaning "paste" or "dough," is a staple in Italian restaurants. Pasta is basically created from flour (sometimes durum and sometimes all-purpose flour), water, and/or eggs. These ingredients are used to create a wide variety of different pastas, from angel hair to ziti.

Unlike Italy of yesterday, you see many differently colored and spiced pastas in American restaurants today. There are whole-wheat, tomato, spinach, artichoke, and many more types of pastas. It's hard to decipher all the shapes and names of pastas used today. Here is a basic primer to help you "Know Your Pastas" and have an easier time deciding which one to order.

Agnolotti–crescent-shaped pieces of pasta, stuffed with one ingredient or a combination of cheese, meat, and spinach.

Angel hair–the thinnest and finest of the "long" pasta family, it is quite light in consistency and often served with light sauces.

Cannelloni–large, tubular pasta, similar to manicotti, it is stuffed with one ingredient or a combination of cheese, meat, and spinach.

Capellitti—meaning a "little hat," these are small, stuffed pastas that look like little tortellini; often stuffed with cheese or meats.

Fettucini—flat, long noodle about ¼-inch wide (wider than linguine).

Fusilli—spiral-shaped long pasta, fusilli is round like spaghetti.

Gnocchi—little dumplings, in ½-inch pieces made from either flour, potato, or a combination of both; often topped with sauce.

Lasagne—the widest noodle among the long, flat pastas; found with either smooth or scalloped edges.

Linguine—flat, long noodle about ⅛-inch wide (thinner than fettucini).

Manicotti—long, tubular noodle about 2 inches in diameter, most often stuffed with cheese and/or meat and served with tomato sauce.

Mostaccioli—short, tubular noodle about 1½ inches long

Penne—short, tubular noodle quite similar to mostaccioli and rigatoni.

Polenta—corn meal and water mixture, which is cooked, poured on a board to harden, and served with a sauce.

Ravioli—pasta about 2 inches square, with corrugated edges, always stuffed with cheese, spinach, or meats in combination or singly.

Rigatoni—short, tubular noodle quite similar to penne and mostaccioli.

Risotto—Italian short-grain rice that has a creamy consistency when cooked; often mixed with butter and cheese before serving.

Shells—noodles in the shape of conch shells, called *conchiglie* in Italian, and found in a variety of sizes; sometimes larger ones are stuffed, and most are served topped with tomato sauce.

Spaghetti—thin, round pasta (also called vermicelli); the most commonly known pasta in America.

Tortelini—small pastas, stuffed and joined at the ends to form a ring: a larger version of capellitti.

Ziti—a short, tubular pasta similar to mostaccioli.

8

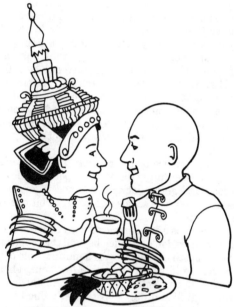

Healthier eating out
Thai Style

Most Americans are familiar with the Chinese menu entries of egg roll, chow mein, or moo shi but much less familiar with tod mun, shrimp choo chee, or pad thai, the listings frequently seen in a Thai restaurant. However, Americans recently have and will continue to become more familiar with these Thai menu regulars. In a few years the Thai soup—tom yum koong will be as well known as won ton.

Over the last five to ten years, there has been an onslaught of Thai restaurants opening around the country, especially in the large cities. A recent cooking magazine calls Thai food "the newest cuisine we've imported from the Orient. It's aromatic Thai, with trim vegetables, light sauces and seasonings that tingle and tantalize." The author, William Clifford, adds that "some people have wondered if Thai food is only the latest Oriental fad, or whether its unique flavoring will ensure its place on America's international menu. The recent proliferation of Thai restaurants indicates that . . . Thai cooking is here to stay."

Beyond simply our yen for great hot and spicy Thai foods is an increasing knowledge that our eating habits must be modified to improve our health status. Thai food, generally speaking, fits into the healthy goals for eating—light on the fats, meats, and sauces and heavy on the vegetables, noodles, and rice. Overall, Thai food may well be a healthier choice than Chinese food, the cuisine with which it's frequently compared.

Because there are more and more Thai restaurants popping up, seemingly daily, more people are trying Thai food and going back for seconds. Many people agree that Thai food seems lighter and a bit healthier than Chinese food.

Thai cuisine is often compared with Chinese though the similarities don't go much beyond the preparation technique of stir-frying, the predominant role of rice, and using similar ingredients—a few being shrimp, chicken, onions, and mushrooms. As far as end results, Thai food differs substantially due to many different spicing agents. In fact, taste-wise, Thai food more closely resembles Indian fare. India and China are both Thailand's neighbors, so it's easy to see why both countries, as well as other Southeast Asian lands, have influenced Thai cooking.

Both Indian and Thai cuisine have hot and spicy qualities as well as what's often called an aromatic flavor. These qualities are achieved through the use of spices—coriander, cumin, cardamom, cinnamon, and several others. These are blended to develop what Americans know as a curry flavor. The use of chilies, which pack a bit of punch, is also a similarity. The use of tamarind, tumeric, and coconut milk is also reminiscent of India.

But, interestingly, the manner in which foods are cut up into small pieces and quickly cooked by stir-frying in a wok more closely resembles Thailand's eastern neighbor, China, than the Indian style of stewing. Some people say there are even Malaysian influences in Thai cooking. The frequently offered appetizer, satay, has its roots in Malaysian cooking techniques.

Thai cuisine, with its many influences, certainly has its unique light flavors and spices. Thais use nam pla, or fish sauce, similarly to the way Chinese use soy sauce, though soy sauce is also frequently used in Thai cooking. Several different pastes—dried fish and spice combinations such as shrimp paste, or kapi—are used to flavor dishes. Lemon grass (takrai), kaffir lime leaves (makrut), and basil (horapa) are somewhat unique, commonly used Thai spices. See "Spices, Seasonings, and Ingredients of Thai Cuisine" at the end of the chapter for further details. You'll also taste the familiar ginger and garlic, which is consistent with other Southeast Asian cuisines.

Thai cooking techniques, mainly done quickly and on top of the stove, do use fat. Some fried appetizers and main entrees appear on most menus. It's easier to skirt the fried entrees than the appetizers, most of which are fried. However, deep frying is by no means the most frequently used cooking method. Most often, dishes are stir-fried, steamed, boiled, or barbecued. Fats, as usual, are used in the cooking vessel, the wok.

In Thailand, it's typical to use lard or coconut oil in cooking. Both contain saturated fat, and lard, being an animal fat, contains cholesterol. I spoke with several Thai restaurateurs who, when asked, said they use vegetable oil for stir-frying. Hopefully, this is or will eventually be true for all Thai restaurants. A positive factor of Thai dishes is that sauces are very light and flavorful. They're not as heavy as the familiar oyster and black bean sauce of Chinese cooking. One reason for this is that little or no thickening agents, such as flour or cornstarch, are added to Thai dishes.

Coconut milk is used in substantial volume in Thai cuisine, and, unfortunately, similar to coconut oil the milk is loaded with calories and saturated fat. In fact, according to the USDA nutrient analysis, a cup of canned coconut milk contains 445 calories, about 97 percent of which are fat. There are certain dishes to navigate around, such as the coconut-milk laden curry entrees, when enjoying Thai food.

Rice, as is common in many Southeast Asian countries, is a staple in Thailand. It's always served at the main meals. The rice most frequently used is a long-grain white rice. Interestingly, no salt is added when preparing rice according to Thai customs. Fried rice (one popular variety is called mee grub) and noodles (one famous version is known as pad thai) are familiar starches in Thailand.

Traditionally, a main meal in Thailand consists of soup, rice, a curry dish, assorted vegetables, a salad, and several sauces. As in Indian style, it is common and quite acceptable for people to eat with their fingers. However, chopsticks are used, and in certain parts of Thailand the fork and spoon are employed. Knives aren't often used because foods are in small pieces and don't need to be cut further.

How foods look seems just as important as how they taste. It's important that dishes are aesthetically pleasing. In Thai restaurants time is taken to carve fruits and vegetables and place them on serving platters to please the eyes of the diner. You might also see flowers and leaves used to decorate tables and serving plates.

Though there are some Thai foods and preparation methods one should avoid, there are many, many palate-pleasing entries on Thai menus. In addition, sharing dishes is the way most people enjoy Thai cuisine. That style makes portion control easier and allows you to taste a wider variety of menu selections.

What to consider before ordering

Generally due to its lighter qualities, Thai food can be quite a healthy choice for people monitoring their consumption of fats, cholesterol, and sugar. If smart menu choices are selected, Thai cuisine can nicely match the nutrition goals for healthy eating. Whether heart disease, diabetes, or just general health maintenance is your concern, Thai food might expand the horizon of ethnic cuisines you enjoy.

When observing the menu to make your selections, keep close tabs on the number of chili symbols, asterisks, or other notations alongside particular dishes. These indicate the hot and spicy quality of the dish. Three notations usually means you'd better have a glass of water poured and within reach. If you see a dish that appeals to you yet you think it will be either too spicy or not hot enough, just ask the waitperson to request that the chef turn the punch up or down. Don't forget, though, that the punch basically is contributed by spices and flavorings that have no calories or fat—so go ahead and be daring!

Due to the predominant role rice plays as a staple in the Thai diet, it's easy to keep the carbohydrates up. Another help in boosting carbos is that it's easy to find dishes that incorporate vegetables. You'll see dishes that combine four, five, or six different vegetables. And there are always a few vegetarian menu offerings. It's easy to keep the meat, poultry, or seafood portions down, especially if you order a dish that contains many vegetables. It's much easier to eat less than four to five ounces of protein in a Thai restaurant than it is in an American steak house or hamburger joint.

The most common protein foods listed on the menu are seafood—shrimp, scallops, squid, and clams. It's not uncommon to see several seafood combination dishes. You'll also see plenty of chicken and duck entries. Duck is best to avoid due to its high fat content, and it's often seen fried on Thai menus. If it's sliced duck with no skin, that's fine on occasion. In addition, beef and pork are the focus of many dishes. Both are fine choices as long as they are mixed with vegetables and balanced with seafood or vegetable dishes as the second or third entree ordered for group sharing.

As previously mentioned, traditionally Thais use some saturated fats in their cooking. It's possible that lard or coconut oil is used in the wok. So be sure to ask what type of fats are used. If the response is lard or coconut oil, try requesting that vegetable oil be used to prepare your dishes. If the request is made often enough by concerned diners, the restaurant will eventually change the fat they use. And remember, vegetable oil doesn't decrease the calories, just the saturated fat and, in the case of lard, the cholesterol.

As for limiting your fat consumption, keep an eye out for the Red Flag Words, most of which indicate that fat has been used. Fried, deep-fried, and crisp are telltale signs that you should move on to another choice. To minimize fat, look for the stir-fried, steamed, sauteed, boiled, marinated, grilled, and barbecued menu listings.

Another way to stay low on fats is to watch out for dishes that mention coconut milk or cream. Coconut milk is found in some soups as well as in entrees. The description of the item usually denotes the addition of coconut milk. Curry dishes seem to contain large amounts of coconut milk and might best be avoided if saturated fat is a big concern. If you eat a small quantity, and don't eat Thai food all that often, a bit of coconut milk once in a while is not really a problem. Certainly try to avoid it as best you can. One positive attribute of coconut milk is that it has almost no sodium.

The sodium content of Thai food is not as great as it often is in Japanese food, but certainly it can still run high. The spicing and flavoring of Thai food is not as dependent on soy sauces as the other Oriental cuisines. However, it is not uncommon to see soy sauce and/or salt added to main dishes, soups, rice, and noodle dishes (other than steamed rice). Some of the sauces, such as yellow bean paste, shrimp paste, and fish sauce, add some sodium.

It's best, as usual, to avoid the soups if you've been encouraged to keep sodium on the low side. You can certainly try requesting that less salt and/or soy be used in preparing your dishes. Also, to minimize sodium a bit more, request that no MSG be used. On average, a rough estimate is that entree servings will have 400–600 milligrams of sodium. Obviously, the more you eat, the more sodium you consume.

People with diabetes should be advised that, in similar fashion to many Southeast Asian cuisines, a small amount of sugar is used in many dishes. Sometimes Thais use palm sugar. If you feel that even a small amount of sugar makes your blood sugar rise, ask that the sugar be left out when the dish is prepared. On average, one teaspoon to two tablespoons of sugar might be added to a whole dish. If you use the recipe guideline discussed in the June, 1989 issue of *Diabetes Forecast* that no more than one teaspoon of sugar be used per serving, then most Thai recipes will be fine. It's important to skirt sweet-and-sour dishes, other dishes that are described as being sweet, and desserts other than fruits.

Managing the menu

Most of the appetizers are simply off limits if you're closely monitoring fat and calories. Consider the common fried listings of Thai rolls, tod mun, fried or stuffed chicken wings, and golden bags. Some of the portions are small, and if you've got a few more calories to spare, then limit yourself to splitting one appetizer or eating one piece of an appetizer if you're dining with a group. A couple of healthier appetizer choices frequently found on Thai menus are satay and steamed mussels. Both of these are an improvement over the fried choices. If your dining partner is also interested in eating healthier, you might just dive right into the main entrees and skip the appetizers.

Another option, rather than skipping right to the main course, is to stop by the soups. Again, soups can be filling and take the edge off a voracious appetite. Thai soups seem to break into two clear categories: healthy choices and ones to avoid. There are several broth-based soups, such as tom yum koong and pok taek, that have a bit of protein and great taste derived from the usual Thai spices of lemon grass, chili paste, and lime juice. These have a low calorie count. However, as usual with soup, they're high in sodium. The soups to avoid, due to the added coconut milk, are tom ka gai, or chicken coconut soup. You simply have to read the description of the item to determine whether the base is made with coconut milk.

Thai restaurants consistently have several salads listed on the menu. Salads are somewhat unusual in Southeast Asian cuisines but seem to be a staple in Thai cookery. That's great news for those interested in eating healthy. Thai salads range from simple garden salads with mainly vegetables to beef, chicken, and seafood, or combinations such as yam yai that mixes shrimp, chicken, and pork. What's great is that the dressings are light and made with Thai spices— lemon grass, chili, lime juice, and sometimes peanut sauce. Go ahead and ask to have the dressing on the side, as usual, so you can control how much goes on the salad. Think about using the Thai garden salad as an appetizer if others are indulging in greasy appetizers. Or order a salad as your main course with a bowl of rice; or split the salad with your dining partner(s). A little roughage always helps fill you up and not out.

Among the entrees you'll find many healthy choices. There are many selections that are loaded with vegetables and cooked in light sauces. So think about which protein foods you want—chicken, shrimp, scallops, fish, beef, or pork, and then find a dish that suits your fancy. Think about complementing a protein-filled dish with a vegetable or a vegetable and tofu (bean curd) mixture. This helps keep the carbos up and the protein down. As usual, look out for the Red Flag Words: fried, deep fried, crispy, and until golden brown should raise the warning signal that fat is in your midst. Compare the unhealthy and healthy sound of the following two dishes: pla Jean – deep fried fish topped with onions, ginger, scallions, black mushroom, and popcorn shrimp vs. poy sian – seafood sauteed with straw mushrooms, napa, bamboo shoots, baby corn, onions, and string peas.

It's not uncommon to see peanuts, cashews, or peanut sauces used in Thai cooking. It's easy enough to request that nuts be left off if you like the rest of the contents of the dish. If calories are a big concern, the lighter basil, chili, lime juice, and Thai spice sauces might be better choices and are easy enough to find.

The curry dishes that are almost always found on Thai menus add quite a bit of coconut milk. They often state "Made with coconut milk" in the description. If saturated fat and calories are big concerns, it might be best to steer away from the curry dishes. However, if you order one curry dish to share among two or more and make an effort not to use too much sauce, the curry dishes can be fine choices. They often have lots of vegetables included. In most places you can get vegetable or tofu curry. They contain no meats or seafood. You can often choose from red, green, yellow, mussaman curry, and more. These describe different curry mixtures and the color of certain spices used.

Several rice and noodle offerings appear on the menu. Hands down, the best choice, which often comes automatically with entrees, is steamed white rice. Traditionally, no salt or fat is added in cooking. You can't beat it for healthfulness. Fried rice choices are often available, either vegetable, pork, seafood, or fried rice combinations. No question, you up the sodium and fat content when you move from white to fried. But if you've got a few calories to spare, you might want to try some of each.

The most common Thai noodle dish is pad Thai. It consists of noodles stir-fried with ground peanuts, bean sprouts, egg, tofu, and scallions and usually served with a few shrimp on top. It's great but certainly has more fat and sodium than steamed white rice. Again, have a small portion but also have the steamed white rice. There are several other noodle dishes. They usually contain a combination of small amounts of protein foods, such as shrimp, egg, and vegetables, that are all stir-fried together with some Thai spices added.

The dessert listings in most Thai restaurants are minimal and best passed by. There is little attention given to dessert. You might find lychee nuts, a common Southeast Asian fruit, and puddings or custards listed. The lychee nuts are fine, but you might just want to enjoy a nice, relaxing cup of coffee or tea or a glass of mineral water.

When the menu arrives, look for certain key words and phrases that signal the nutritional advisability of the items. We call them "Green Flag" (go for it) and "Red Flag" (steer clear) words.

Green Flag Words

stir-fried
sauteed
sizzling
broiled, boiled, or steamed
braised,
marinated
barbecued
charbroiled
basil sauce, basil, or sweet basil leaves
lime sauce or lime juice
chili sauce or crushed dried chili
Thai spices
served in a hollowed-out pineapple
fish sauce
hot sauce
napa, bamboo shoots, black mushrooms, ginger, garlic
bed of mixed vegetables
scallions, onions

sizzling deep-fried
fried
deep-fried
crispy
until golden brown
stir-fried

**Red Flag
Words**
topped with peanuts, peanut sauce
peanuts, cashews
curry sauce (often made with lots
   of coconut milk)
made with coconut milk
eggplant (most often fried)
golden brown duck

Please hold the peanuts (or
   cashews) from this dish.
Can you prepare these dishes
   with no MSG?
What oil is used to prepare your
   foods? (If it's coconut oil or lard,

**Special
Requests
Thai
Style**
   ask that vegetable oil be used
   instead.)
Please minimize the salt and soy
   sauce; I'm carefully watching
   my sodium consumption.
Can I substitute scallops for
   shrimp or beef in this dish?
Could I have a bit more broccoli
   and less beef in this dish?
Could I get the rest of this
   wrapped up to take home; I'd
   like to enjoy it for dinner tomorrow night?
Please put the dressing on the
   side of the salad.
Please make this dish equivalent
   to three-chili hotness; I like lots
   of flavor.

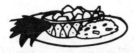

Typical Menu: Thai Style

Appetizers   **Thai rolls** (delicate and crispy vegetable-filled spring rolls served with sweet-and-sour sauce)

✓**Satay** (beef or chicken marinated in coconut milk and curry, barbecued on skewers, and served with peanut sauce and cucumber salad)

Tod mun (minced shrimp and codfish, mixed wth Thai curry, and fried until golden brown; served with cucumber sauce)

✓**Steamed mussels** (steamed with lemon grass, sweet basil leaves, chili, and Thai spices; served with chili sauce)

✓**Seafood kebab** (shrimp, scallops, and vegetables on skewers, served with hot sauce)

Vegetarian tofu (deep-fried tofu served with sweet chili sauce)

Soups   ✓**Tom yum koong** (Thai shrimp soup with lemon grass, chili paste, lime juice, and straw mushrooms)

Tom ka gai (chicken in coconut milk soup with mushrooms and lime juice)

✓**Crystal noodle** (clear soup with chicken, bean thread noodles, and vegetables)

✓**Talay thong** (seafood combination with chili, lemon grass, basil leaves, and snow peas)

✓**Pok taek** (shrimp, squid, scallops, mushrooms with lemon grass, chili paste, and lime juice)

✓*Preferred Choice*

Salads   ✓**Thai salad** (green mixed garden
salad with tofu and egg wedges,
dressed with spiced peanut sauce)

✓**Pla koong** (spicy shrimp salad
with onion, scallions, tomatoes,
mushrooms, lemon grass, all
tossed with chili and lime juice)

✓**Spiced beef salad** (charbroiled
beef slices in chili paste, lemon
grass, lettuce, tomatoes,
mushrooms, and scallions tossed
in spicy lemon dressing)

✓**Yam yai** (spicy combination salad
of shrimp, pork, and chicken with
lettuce, cucumber, onion, and
tomato in light Thai spicy
dressing)

Curry   The following curry dishes can be
made with either chicken, beef,
shrimp, scallops, tofu, or
vegetables.

✓**Green curry** (in coconut milk,
with bamboo shoots, green peppers, string beans, green peas,
and zucchini)

✓**Red curry** (in coconut milk, with
bamboo shoots, red and green
peppers)

✓**Yellow** (in coconut milk, with
potatoes, onion, green pepper, and
summer squash)

✓**Mussaman curry** (in coconut
milk, with potatoes, onions, carrots, and peanuts)

Poultry   **Crispy duck** (fried duck, steamed
with soy sauce, topped with fried
spinach, and served with plum
sauce)

√**Thai chicken** (chicken sauteed with cashews, onions, mushrooms, pineapple, scallions, and chili; served in a whole pineapple)

Chicken in the garden (boiled, sliced chicken on a bed of broccoli, carrots, cauliflower, green beans, and asparagus; topped with peanut sauce)

√**Sweet-and-sour chicken** (slices of chicken, pineapple, tomatoes, onions, and green peppers topped with a sweet-and-sour sauce)

√**Chili duck** (sauteed roast duck with onion, hot pepper, mushrooms, scallions, and fresh sweet basil leaves with spiced tomato sauce)

Beef/Pork　　**Spareribs curry** (red curry in coconut milk, with boneless spareribs, peas, string beans, snowpeas, hot pepper, tomato, and sweet basil leaves)

√**Beef basil** (sauteed beef flavored with hot basil leaves, fresh hot pepper, mushrooms, and red pepper)

√**Pork and string beans** (sauteed sliced pork tenderloin with string beans, snowpeas, red pepper, and cashew nuts tossed in spicy chili sauce)

Praram long song (fried beef with special curry sauce and peanuts over a bed of spinach)

√**Chili beef** (sauteed sliced beef with baby corn, onions, mushrooms, and red and green peppers topped with chili sauce)

√**Ginger pork** (sauteed pork in ginger with green pepper, onion, scallion, mushrooms, and chili paste)

Seafood   **Hot Thai catfish** (deep-fried catfish fillet topped with bamboo
shoots, baby corn, mushrooms,
eggplant, hot chili, and basil
leaves with Thai spices)

✓**Garlic shrimp** (sauteed shrimp
with fresh garlic, peppercorns,
snowpeas, and napa; served on a
bed of sliced cucumbers)

✓**Poy sian** (combination of seafood
sauteed with straw mushrooms,
napa, bamboo shoots, onions, and
string beans)

✓**Scallops bamboo** (sauteed sea
scallops, with bamboo shoots,
snowpeas, baby corn, mushrooms,
and scallions all mixed with Thai
spices)

✓**Seafood platter** (sauteed assorted
seafood, shrimp, scallops, squid,
and clams, with celery, baby corn,
and onions and a yellow bean
sauce)

Vegetables   **Royal tofu** (deep-fried pieces of
tofu with snowpeas, onions, scal-
lions, and broccoli seasoned with
a spicy chili sauce)

✓**Vegetable boat** (string beans,
asparagus, zucchini, onions, and
mushrooms stir-fried in Thai
spices)

✓**Pad jay** (combination of napa,
celery, onions, carrots,
mushrooms, and bean sprouts
topped with a sauce of Thai
spices)

Rice and Noodles	**Fried rice** (rice fried with chicken, scallions, green peas, onion, and egg) **Vegetable fried rice** (rice fried with assorted stir-fry vegetables) ✓**Steamed rice** ✓**Pad Thai** (noodles stir-fried with ground peanuts, bean sprouts, egg, tofu, and scallions, topped with shrimp)
Desserts	✓**Lychee nuts** **Fried banana** (deep-fried banana served with a sweet syrup sauce) **Tapioca** (coconut pudding) **Thai custard**

Now that you've seen what may be available on the menu, look over the following five "Model Meals" for suggestions on how to order to achieve specific nutrition goals. Models are numbered one to five for quick reference, and each is followed by an "Estimated Nutrient Evaluation" that analyzes the content of that meal.

May I Take Your Order

Healthy	30% Calories as fat
Daily	20% Calories as protein
Eating	50% Calories as carbohydrate
Goals	300 mg/day Cholesterol
	3000 mg/day Sodium

Low Calorie/ **Tom yum koong**
Low Fat *Quantity:* 1 cup
Model Meal *Exchanges:* ½ meat; ½ vegetable
Thai chicken (hold cashews)
Quantity: 1 cup
Exchanges: 2 meat (lean); 1 fat;
  1 vegetable
Poy sian
Quantity: 1 cup
Exchanges: 2 meat (lean); 1 fat;
  1 vegetable
Steamed rice
Quantity: 1 cup
Exchanges: 3 starch
Mineral water
Quantity: 12 oz
Exchanges: free

Estimated	528 calories
Nutrient	29% calories as fat
Evaluation	22% calories as protein
	49% calories as carbohydrate
	153 mg cholesterol
	1210 mg sodium

❷

Low Calorie/
Low
Cholesterol
Model Meal

Pok taek
Quantity: 1 cup
Spiced beef salad
Quantity: 2 cups
Steamed rice
Quantity: 1 cup
Hot tea
Quantity: 2 cups

Estimated
Nutrient
Evaluation

593 calories
32% calories as fat
27% calories as protein
41% calories as carbohydrate
100 mg cholesterol
1069 mg sodium

❸

Higher
Calorie/Low
Fat Model
Meal

Green curry with tofu
Quantity: 1½ cups
Exchanges: 2 fat; 3 vegetable
Scallops bamboo
Quantity: 1½ cups
Exchanges: 3 meat (lean); 1 fat; 2
vegetable
Pad Thai
Quantity: 1 cup
Exchanges: ½ meat (lean); 2 fat; 2
starch
Steamed rice
Quantity: ⅔ cup
Exchanges: 2 starch
Coffee
Quantity: 2 cups
Exchanges: free

Estimated
Nutrient
Evaluation

818 calories
35% calories as fat
23% calories as protein
42% calories as carbohydrate
64 mg cholesterol
1260 mg sodium

❹
Higher Calorie/Low Cholesterol Model Meal

Satay, chicken
Quantity: 2 skewers
Ginger pork
Quantity: 1½ cups
Vegetable boat
Quantity: 1½ cups
Fried rice with vegetables
Quantity: 1⅓ cups
Light beer
Quantity: 12 oz

Estimated Nutrient Evaluation

976 calories
38% calories as fat
20% calories as protein
34% calories as carbohydrate
8% calories as alcohol
136 mg cholesterol
1460 mg sodium

❺
Low Sodium Model Meal

Yam yai salad
Quantity: 1½ cups
Sweet-and-sour chicken
Quantity: 1½ cups
Steamed rice
Quantity: 1 cup
White wine
Quantity: 6 oz

Estimated Nutrient Evaluation

781 calories
24% calories as fat
24% calories as protein
37% calories as carbohydrate
15% calories as alcohol
138 mg cholesterol
820 mg sodium

Spices, seasonings, and ingredients of Thai cuisine

Bamboo shoots—an oriental vegetable commonly found in Thai entrees; light in color, crunchy, and stringy in texture and very low in calories.

Basil—*horapa*, as it's known in Thailand, basil is used mainly in leaf form; there are several types of basil used in Thai cooking.

Cardamom—a member of the ginger family, the seeds are often used in curry mixtures and other dishes, as seeds or ground.

Chilies—various types used, depending on hotness of dish; red and green are common, used whole, chopped, or ground into paste for sauces.

Coconut milk—liquid extracted from grating fresh coconut, not the liquid from inside the coconut; used in marinating and in gravies for various dishes, especially curry sauces.

Coriander—dried coriander seed is the main ingredient in curry mixtures; the seeds or leaves are used; an essential spice in Thai cooking.

Cumin—another fragrant spice important to curry mixtures, used either as seeds or ground.

Curry—really a combination of spices, not a single spice as known in the U.S.; different spice and food combinations create the green, red, and mussaman curry mixtures.

Kapi—dried shrimp paste made from prawns or shrimp, commonly used to flavor many Thai dishes.

Lemon grass—*takrai*, as it's known in Thailand, is an Asian plant whose bulbous base is used to add a lemony flavor to many soups and main entrees.

Lime—*makrut*, in Thai, lime leaves or the juice of kaffir lime is commonly used in soups, salads, and entrees.

Nam pla—a fish sauce used like soy sauce in Thai cooking; this thin, salty brown sauce brings out the flavor of other foods.

Thai Style

Nam prik—called Thai shrimp sauce, it is used to flavor many Thai foods; made from shrimp paste, chilies, lime juice, soy sauce, and sugar.

Napa—also referred to as Chinese cabbage, it has thick-ribbed stalks and crinkled leaves.

Palm sugar—a strong-flavored, dark sugar obtained from the sap of coconut palms; it is boiled down until it crystallizes.

Scallions—also called spring onions, they are white, slender, and have long green stems; usually they are chopped into small pieces.

Soy sauce—used in many Thai dishes to cast a salty flavor; made from soy beans.

Tamarind—an acidy-tasting fruit from a large tropical tree; used for its acid flavor.

Tumeric—the spice that lends the yellow-orange color to commercial curry; part of the ginger family.

9

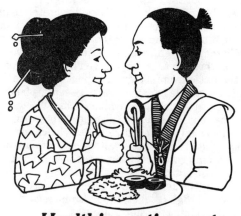

Healthier eating out
Japanese Style

When Japanese food is mentioned, many people form images of meals at Japanese steak houses. These so-called Japanese, but relatively Americanized, restaurants serve the familiar tempura, sukiyaki, and teriyaki. There's usually a talented Japanese chef cooking or, more correctly, performing in front of you. My most vivid memory of these meals is the flying shrimp that somehow land in the center of each person's plate. These restaurants still abound in many large cities. However, there are many smaller, more authentic Japanese restaurants regularly serving such foreign-sounding items as agemono, yosenabe, and donburi. Along with the many cooked entrees, there's usually an assortment of sushi and sashimi available.

As more and more people who eat out search for healthier foods, authentically prepared Japanese food is gaining in popularity. Japanese food is one of the healthiest ethnic cuisines. It's heavy on vegetables, white rice, and seafood and light on meats, dairy products, and fats. The biggest health concern in eating Japanese meals is their high sodium content from all the soy-based sauces.

When you first pick up a Japanese menu and begin learning about the restaurant's offerings, you might feel terribly confused; but it's really quite simple. You'll quickly understand the words that mean chicken, broiled, steamed, and so on, because they frequently reappear and are defined on menus. Even as you read through this chapter, you'll begin to recognize the basic terminology of Japanese cuisine.

Japanese people in Japan are, in general, a healthy population, suffering less frequently than Westerners from the obesity-induced diseases. Interestingly, epidemiological studies have traced the changes in eating habits relative to health status of Japanese who have emigrated from Japan to the United States over the last few decades. It should come as no surprise that as the Japanese immigrants adopted a more Westernized high-fat diet, they also increased their risk of developing Western diseases.

People began emigrating from Japan to the U.S. in the mid-1800s, but by the 1920s this immigration was halted. There was another large influx of Japanese into the U.S. after World War II. There are now a huge number of individuals of Japanese descent in America. The majority of Japanese-Americans continue to live in Hawaii and on the West Coast.

Though Japanese food preparation and presentation at first glance seem quite unique, some of the origins can be traced to Chinese roots. Certain similarities are apparent in the core foods of both countries—rice, soy products, and tea. There are some European influences on Japanese cooking style as well. For instance, the original idea for the familiar tempura has its roots in Portuguese cuisine. It is said that the Japanese learned how to make a much lighter and almost translucent batter. The Japanese dish tonkatsu, which translates into fried pork cutlet, is said to imitate the German dish Wiener schnitzel. Again the Japanese interpretation is lighter and more delicate.

Though there are Asian and European influences on Japanese cuisine, it remains a rather unique style of cookery and meal service. Japanese cookery was described as "making the most of nature's seasonal offerings with utmost culinary artistry" by Shizuo Tsuji, the author of *Japanese Cooking, A Simple Art*.

Food in the Japanese culture does more than simply nourish the body. Importance is placed on the harmony of foods and the role food plays in fueling the body as well as the soul. It is extremly important that foods are served in an aesthetically pleasing manner. You only have to observe people making sushi to appreciate the culinary artistry of Japanese foods. The raw fish, often rolled and served over sushi rice, is cut and placed in creative ways. It's then served on decorative plates, with the side items of shoyu and wasabi and possibly grated carrots aesthetically arranged in the lacquered bowl. The result is almost too beautiful to eat.

Many different-sized plates, bowls, and sauce dishes are used to please the Japanese diner's eye rather than the palate. Boxes, called *bentos,* are sometimes used to serve Japanese meals. Soups are often served in china or lacquered bowls with covers to retain the heat. Beyond the accent placed on the harmony between the food and serving pieces, the physical surroundings also receive attention.

In addition to aesthetics, Japanese cookery is based in simplicity, purity, and sparseness of seasonings. It has evolved as a very light, delicate, and healthy cuisine. There are only a few basic ingredients, and they find their way into most appetizers, soups, salads, and main courses.

Soybeans, and the products that result from their processing, are central to Japanese cooking. Tofu, soy bean curd, is considered an important protein food in the Japanese diet. Soy beans are also the base for shoyu, the Japanese soy sauce. Miso, the fermented soy bean paste, is used in soups and entrees. Teriyaki sauce, which is almost as familiar to Americans as apple pie, also has its base in soy beans. Teriyaki sauce is a combination of shoyu and mirin (sweet rice wine).

Rice, called *gohan,* is a staple in Japan. It's eaten at almost every meal. Rice is also the base of several other predominantly used ingredients in Japanese cookery, including mirin, sake, and Japanese rice vinegar.

Due to the fact that Japan is surrounded by water, fish and shellfish have been major protein sources in the Japanese diet. Poultry is used but less frequently than seafood. Beef and pork, due to their expense and scarcity, were not commonly used, a fact you might not realize when reading a Japanese menu in America. The poultry and beef selections appear just as predominantly as the seafood offerings.

Along with rice, vegetables contribute to the lightness of Japanese cuisine. It's common to find vegetables such as bamboo shoots, napa, mushrooms, scallions, and onions included in Japanese dishes. These are similar vegetables to those found in many Chinese dishes. It is also common to see pickled vegetables on Japanese menus. Pickling was used as a method of preservation prior to the days of refrigeration.

Similar to many Southeast Asian cuisines, there is little or no use of dairy products. You don't see milk, cream, yogurt, or cheeses. Many claim that is true because many Southeast Asians are lactose intolerant, meaning they can't properly digest lactose, the milk sugar.

Nori, wakame, and kombu (also spelled konbu) are certainly foreign ingredients to most Americans, but they are very common items in Japanese cooking. They are all seaweeds. Kombu is used in making dashi, the soup stock, and nori is the seaweed used in rolling and forming maki sushi, or rice rolls. There are many other flavoring agents used, such as wasabi and bonito (fish) flakes. See "Seasonings, Spices, and Terms of Japanese Cuisine" at the end of the chapter. The prominent use of seaweed well illustrates the constraints of Japan's once very limited and narrow food supply. Everything possible, including seaweed, was converted into available foods.

Minimal ingredients for seasoning and simple cooking techniques define Japanese cookery. Dashi, the basic soup stock; shoyu, the Japanese soy sauce; miso, the fermented soy bean paste; and mirin, the sweet rice wine, are the main seasoning ingredients. One or more of these are used to provide the flavor of soups, teriyaki and sukiyaki sauces, and many other dishes. On the downside, however, is the fact that most sauces are quite high in sodium, which makes a Japanese meal quite high in sodium, too. Observe the sodium content of the model meals toward the end of the chapter.

Beyond the use of healthy ingredients, the Japanese complete the preparation by using very healthy cooking techniques. Very little fat is incorporated into cooking. It's common to see foods broiled, grilled, boiled, steamed, braised, or simmered. None of these cooking methods introduce much fat. It's also common to see foods pickled or simply served raw, as are sushi and sashimi. Rarely, other than in tempura and agemono preparation methods, are foods fried. The common Chinese and Thai cooking method of stir-frying with oil in a wok is not used in Japan. However, there are several so-called *nabemonos,* or one-pot meals that are often cooked at the table. Sukiyaki, yosenabe, and shabu-shabu fall into this category.

In Japan the dinner meal usually includes rice (of course), a soup, and pickled vegetables. The main dish most often is fish or shellfish that has been broiled, steamed, or dried. Traditionally, all the dishes are presented at the same time. If any item is held back, it might be the soup, which is served at the end of the meal. This is in contrast to the way Japanese meals are served in the U.S. They have bent toward our custom of serving the appetizer first, then soup, followed by rice and the main course(s). Notice that there is very little focus on dessert.

What to consider before ordering

Japanese foods, preparation, and style of eating represent one of the healthiest ways to enjoy dining out. The cuisine accents the carbohydrates in rice and vegetables and minimizes fats by using food preparation methods that require little or no oil or fat. In addition, small portions are the standard in Japanese fare. That works well for the calorie and health-conscious diner. The only drawback to Japanese food, as stated, is the heavy use of high-sodium flavorings and sauces. But with some adaptations, even a person carefully monitoring sodium consumption can enjoy a Japanese meal.

The higher than desirable sodium level of Japanese food is mainly contributed by the soy-based items. Marinades and sauces, whether for teriyaki, sukiyaki, or shabu-shabu, are a combination of some or all of the following: shoyu, dashi, mirin, sugar, sake, and a bit of kombu.

Unfortunately, if you order a dish such as teriyaki, you can be assured that the protein, whether it is meat or fish, has been prepared in the high-sodium sauce. However, if you order a dish such as shabu-shabu, you can closely control the amount of sauce used because this dish is cooked at the table and you do the dipping. Other strategies to reduce sodium include choosing appetizers that are not marinated or cooked in the high-sodium ingredients. Try some steamed items or have sashimi, the raw fish. Avoid as much of the dipping sauce as possible, use it mainly for flavor, and go heavy on the very low-sodium, but punchy, wasabi.

On to the main part of the meal. Have a salad rather than soup, and ask for vinegar or lemon rather than the frequently used miso dressing; you'll consume less sodium. White rice with no salt added is the typical starch offered. Fresh fruit is regularly available, and it has next to no sodium.

Japanese food gets the gold star for being a cuisine that uses minimal fat. The preparation methods of serving raw food, broiling, steaming, simmering, etc., use almost no fat. The only preparation methods to avoid are tempura, agemono, and katsu. Also, as usual, monitor the menu for the Red Flag Words that are often indicative of added fats.

Basically, in a Japanese restaurant the only fat you end up with on your plate is the fat you get from the foods you've chosen. Therefore, ordering fish, shellfish, or poultry, rather than selecting the beef or pork, helps keep the fat count down. The size of the portions, whether it's fish or beef, seems to be more in line with healthy guidelines, too, than a typical American meal. This also assists in keeping the fat, saturated fat, and cholesterol content of the meal down.

If oils are used in Japanese cookery, they're mainly the no-cholesterol varieties. They don't use the large amounts of lard and coconut oil that are prevalent in Thai and Indian cookery, though a bit of lard might be rubbed on a pan before cooking. If oil is used, it will be cottonseed, olive, peanut, or sesame seed oil. Sesame seed oil is used in minimal quantity for its wonderful nutty flavor.

It's typical to see sugar incorporated into Japanese food preparation on a regular basis, as is true in most Southeast Asian cuisines. Sugar is used in almost all the sauces and marinades. Sugar is also found in su, or vinegared rice, used in sushi. Su rice is flavored with vinegar, salt, and sugar. This is misleading on many menus because they just refer to it as vinegared rice. Although this is not a concern for the calorie-conscious diner because calories are minimal, it is a concern for people with diabetes.

In the end, most sauces and dishes won't provide you with more than several teaspoons to a tablespoon of sugar. However, it's important that you recognize that sugar is used in these items and an effort should be made to minimize the amount of sauce and gravy you consume. Dip lightly and don't spoon in lots of gravy from sukiyaki, donburi, or other sauced dishes. Also, sashimi with a side order of rice might be a better bet than sushi, which contains the sugary rice.

The regularly served sushi and sashimi are gaining popularity in the United States. It has become an "in" food in some cities, and "raw bars," which always have a supply of sushi and sashimi, have also become more popular in Japanese as well as seafood dining spots. Certainly, sushi and sashimi have a long heritage in Japanese dining.

There are various types of sushi and many different fish, shellfish, and vegetables are used in its creation. Great importance is placed on the freshness of the fish and the creativity with which these foods are served. The adjective "beautiful," not often used to describe foods, definitely can be used to describe the way sushi and sashimi are served.

Sushi, which is just a general term for a combination of raw seafood and vinegared rice (su), is served in a variety of ways. Either in, around, or under the fish you'll find vinegared rice. Served with sushi are wasabi, a strong, green-color horseradish paste, and a soy-based sauce for dipping. There are four basic types of sushi. Oshi is pressed sushi rice served with a marinated or boiled piece of seafood. Nigiri is one of the more common varieties, in which the vinegared rice is hand-shaped and the fish placed on top. Maki combines sushi rice with fish and both are rolled into a cylinder around the seaweed nori. Chirashi sushi is presented with the rice scattered and the seafood served in or on the sushi rice.

Sashimi is more simply served but with no less attention to freshness and beauty. Sashimi is raw, sliced fish served on small shallow dishes. It's served with a cone of wasabi, grated ginger root and a soy-based dipping sauce. Tuna, salmon, lobster, clams, and bream are commonly used for sashimi.

Calorically speaking, both sushi and sashimi are smart choices if you enjoy raw fish. They can be ordered as an appetizer or used as a main course. If desired, sashimi can be complemented with a bowl of steamed rice and tossed salad with miso dressing; the result is a low-fat and relatively low-sodium meal.

There are some health concerns about eating raw fish. In fact, due to the rise in raw fish being served in the U.S., there has been an increase of fish-borne illnesses. One disease that can develop is anisakiasis. Anisakis is a parasitic roundworm that lives in larval form in fish, most often in the internal organs. On occasion, the roundworms find their way into the flesh of the fish. If the fish is not cleaned well, refrigerated, and cooked properly, in rare instances it can cause severe stomach pain, nausea, and vomiting.

Anisakiasis can result from eating sushi and sashimi because the fish is served raw and the parasite, if present, cannot be killed by the cooking process. Take precaution—if you enjoy these foods, make sure the fish you are eating is fresh, you feel confident that the restaurant serves a lot of it, and it is handled carefully. Interestingly, USDA home economists recommend not eating any raw seafood. For those who want to read more about this concern, a helpful article entitled "When It Comes to Stylish Sushi, It's Safer to Be Square" was printed in *FDA Consumer*, February, 1987.

Managing the menu

There are quite a number of healthy appetizers on most Japanese menus. Firstly, you'll usually find several sushi and sashimi offerings. Other good choices are barbecued, steamed, or pickled items. Many appetizers come with dipping sauces that will often contain shoyu (soy) and small amounts of sugar. If necessary, limit the quantity of sauce used. Avoid the few fried items such as tempura, agetofu (fried bean curd), and fried dumplings.

Light and delicate soups are a mainstay in a Japanese meal. Staying within tradition, soups are found on menus in almost all Japanese restaurants. There is the simple, clear broth called suimono, made with a base of dashi, or bits of vegetables or meats may be added. Any of these are a good, filling start to a Japanese meal. The miso soup, also quite light, might again have a few vegetables and/or pieces of tofu tossed in. The Japanese udon, or noodle soups, will have a few more calories simply from the noodles. They have a dashi base with udon noodles added. Suudon is plain broth with noodles. There are other varieties of udon that have stir-fried beef, vegetables, or tempura items added. It's best to stick with the suudon or yaki-udon.

Salads are usually available in Japanese restaurants. Either tossed green salads, as Americans are used to, tofu, or seafood salads. In Japan, salads are called sunomono or aemono. They are vinegared or otherwise dressed vegetables and seafoods served in small quantities in elegant little bowls. The dressing most commonly encountered in Japanese restaurants in the U.S. is miso, again a combination of the regular Japanese seasonings.

The majority of Japanese entrees are low in fat and potentially low in saturated fat and cholesterol if you choose wisely. There are only a few to steer away from, such as the tempura, agemono, and katsu dishes. Usually there are several styles of food preparation stated on the menu, and the different foods you can have prepared in that fashion are listed underneath. For instance, teriyaki is listed as a preparation category, and you can have chicken, beef, fish, or shellfish prepared in this manner. The same is true for nabemonos, the one-pot meals. Sukiyaki, yosenabi, and shabu-shabu are prominent members of this group.

Nabemonos are better than teriyaki dishes because they have more vegetables and a smaller quantity of protein. However, the technique of sharing again comes in handy. Think about sharing a teriyaki, sukiyaki, or yosenabe order. That way, you'll both have some vegetables and be able to taste two dishes.

Donburi, which reminds me of the Indian dish biryani, is a rice dish topped with broiled or fried meat, fish, or poultry and eggs. It is topped also with a soy-based sauce. Obviously, it's best to have donburi topped with broiled items rather than breaded and fried ones. Donburi, due to the whole eggs used in its preparation, might best be avoided by those carefully monitoring cholesterol. You might ask if eggs can be deleted from the order.

Rice is the staple you'll find automatically served with most dishes. The rice used in Japan is a short-grain variety. It's usually starchier and stickier than the long-grain rice found in Chinese cuisine. It's served plain and blends well with all the sauces and flavors of Japanese foods. Another starch found in Japanese restaurants, but not as predominantly as rice, is noodles. Either udon, wheat noodles, or soba, buckwheat noodles, are sometimes served. Udon noodles are regularly found in the udon soups described previously. Both types of noodles are great—lots of carbos and no fats. Just for variety you might want to try either udon or soba noodles instead of rice.

Dessert in Japan is typically fresh fruit. You'll see a very short list of desserts on most Japanese menus. Restaurants will usually have fresh fruit, ice cream, and maybe yo kan, the sweet bean cake. It's unusual to be able to order fresh fruit at a restaurant, so take advantage of this rare opportunity. At formal dinners, it is customary to serve kashi, or okashi, the Japanese confections.

Green tea and sake are the national beverages of Japan. Tea is drunk just plain—with no sugar, lemon, or milk added. Tea is held in such high esteem in Japan that it has its own ceremony, called *kaiseki,* which is quite an important cultural ritual.

Sake is a fermented beverage, fragrant and colorless. It contains a bit higher alcohol content than most wines, about 15–17 percent. Sake is more often sipped warm than cold. It is served in a sake bottle, *tokkuri,* and poured into individual cups, *sakazuki.*

When the menu arrives, look for certain key words and phrases that signal the nutritional advisability of the items. We call them "Green Flag" (go for it) and "Red Flag" (steer clear) words.

Green Flag Words

steamed (mushimono)
sauteed
clear broth
braised
simmered (nimono)
marinated
vinegared (usually with vinegar,
    salt, and sugar)
seasoned rice
vinegar sauce*
broiled (yaki)
barbecued
grilled (yakimono)
on skewers
teriyaki sauce*
miso*
miso dressing*
dipping sauce*
boiled
served in broth*

*Usually high in sodium content;
    carefully monitor quantity used.

Red Flag Words

deep-fried
tempura
agemono
katsu
battered and fried
fried bean curd
pan-fried
breaded and fried

Special Requests Japanese Style

Could you serve the salad with
    the dressing on the side?
I'm carefully watching my salt in-
    take; can you use less sauce in
    preparing this dish?
Could you substitute shrimp, scal-
    lops, or chicken for the beef in
    this dish?
Could you leave the egg out of the
    sukiyaki (or donburi)?
I couldn't finish all this; may I
    get it wrapped up to take home?

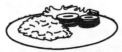

Typical Menu: Japanese Style

Sashimi and Sushi

✓**Sashimi, tuna** (fillet of fresh raw tuna served with wasabi and dipping sauce)

✓**Sashimi, salmon** (fillet of fresh raw salmon served with ginger root and dipping sauce)

✓**Sashimi, combination** (fillet of fresh raw seafood, tuna, salmon, and lobster, with wasabi and dipping sauce)

✓**Chirashi sushi** (fresh raw seafood served on seasoned rice, with pickled vegetables and seaweed)

✓**Maki sushi** (fresh raw tuna and vinegared rice rolled in seaweed)

✓**Sushi combination** (3 nigiri and 3 maki sushi served with wasabi and dipping sauce)

Appetizers

✓**Yutofu** (hot bean curd boiled with napa, served with special sauce)

✓**Ebi-su** (shrimp in vinegar sauce)

✓**Shumai** (steamed shrimp dumplings wrapped in thin noodle skin)

Tempura appetizer (shrimp and vegetables dipped in batter and lightly fried)

✓**Yakitori** (two skewers of chicken broiled with teriyaki sauce)

Agedashi tofu (fried tofu in tempura sauce)

✓**Oshinko** (Japanese pickled vegetables)

✓**Ohitashi** (fresh spinach boiled and served with soy sauce)

✓*Preferred Choice*

Soups	✓**Suimono** (clear broth soup) ✓**Miso** (soy bean paste soup with tofu and scallions) ✓**Su-udon** (plain Japanese noodle soup) **Tempura-udon** (Japanese noodle soup with tempura) ✓**Yaki-udon** (Japanese noodle soup with stir-fried vegetables)
Salads	✓**Tossed salad** served with miso dressing ✓**Tofu salad** served with miso dressing ✓**Seafood sunomono** (seafood with cucumber, seaweed, and shredded garnish with vinegar sauce)

Entrees*	**Tempura** (lightly battered and fried; served with tempura dipping sauce)
	    Shrimp
	    Vegetable
	    Combination shrimp and vegetable
	Teriyaki (broiled and served with teriyaki sauce)
	    ✓Chicken
	    ✓Beef
	    ✓Salmon
	    ✓Seafood combination
	Agemono (battered in breadcrumbs and deep-fried)
	    Tonkatsu (pork cutlet)
	    Chicken katsu
	    Shrimp
	Nabemono (one-pot cooked dinners)
	    ✓Sukiyaki, chicken (sliced chicken, tofu, bamboo shoots, and vegetables simmered in sukiyaki sauce)
	    ✓Sukiyaki, beef (thinly sliced beef, tofu, bamboo shoots, and vegetables simmered in sukiyaki sauce)

    ✓Yosenabe (noodles, seafood,
       and vegetables simmered in
       a special broth)
  ✓**Shabu-shabu** (sliced beef and
  vegetables with noodles cooked
  and served at the table, with dipping sauces)
  Donburi (served on a bed of rice
  with special sauce)
    ✓Oyako (sauteed chicken, egg,
      and onion)
    Katsu (deep-fried breaded pork,
      egg, onion)
    Unagi (broiled eel)

    *Entrees served à la carte with
    steamed white rice or soba
    noodles.

Desserts ✓**Fresh fruit**
        Ice cream, ginger or vanilla
        Yo kan (sweet bean cake)

Now that you've seen what may be available on the
menu, look over the following five "Model Meals" for
suggestions on how to order to achieve specific nutritional goals. Models are numbered one to five for
quick reference, and each is followed by an "Estimated
Nutrient Evaluation" that analyzes the content of
that meal.

May I Take Your Order

Healthy	30% Calories as fat
Daily	20% Calories as protein
Eating	50% Calories as carbohydrate
Goals	300 mg/day Cholesterol
	3000 mg/day Sodium

---

❶

Low Calorie/	**Sashimi, tuna**
Low Fat	*Quantity:* 1 serving
Model Meal	*Exchanges:* 3 meat (lean)
	Dipping sauce for above
	Quantity: 2 tbsp
	Exchanges: free
	Yaki-udon soup
	Quantity: 1 cup
	Exchanges: 1 fat; 1 vegetable; 1 starch
	Steamed rice
	Quantity: 1 cup
	Exchanges: 3 starch
	Tofu salad (dressing on the side)
	Quantity: 1–2 cups
	Exchanges: ½ meat (lean); 1–2 vegetables
	Miso dressing for above (on the side)
	Quantity: 2 tbsp
	Exchanges: free

Estimated	528 calories
Nutrient	16% calories as fat
Evaluation	30% calories as protein
	54% calories as carbohydrate
	76 mg cholesterol
	1490 mg sodium

Low Calorie/ Low Cholesterol Model Meal

Shumai
Quantity: 1 order
Yakitori
Quantity: 2 skewers
Miso soup
Quantity: 1 cup
Steamed rice
Quantity: 1 cup
Tossed salad (dressing on the side)
Quantity: 1–2 cups
Miso dressing for above (on the side)
Quantity: 1–2 tbsp

Estimated Nutrient Evaluation

434 calories
9% calories as fat
31% calories as protein
60% calories as carbohydrate
106 mg cholesterol
1850 mg sodium (lower by using vinegar or lemon wedges on salad)

Higher Calorie/Low Fat Model Meal

Ohitashi
Quantity: 1 order
Exchanges: 1 vegetable
Siumono soup
Quantity: 1 cup
Exchanges: 1 vegetable
Teriyaki, salmon (split order)
Quantity: 4 oz
Exchanges: 4 meat (lean)
Donburi, oyako (split order)
Quantity: 1½ cups
Exchanges: 1 meat (medium); 3 starch

Steamed rice
Quantity: ⅔ cup
Exchanges: 2 starch
Fresh fruit
Quantity: 1 small piece
Exchanges: 1 fruit

Estimated Nutrient Evaluation	
	719 calories
	23% calories as fat
	30% calories as protein
	47% calories as carbohydrate
	251 mg cholesterol (mainly from egg in Donburi)
	1700 mg sodium

❹
Higher Calorie/Low Cholesterol Model Meal

Yutofu
Quantity: 1 order
Su-udon soup
Quantity: 1 cup
Sukiyaki, beef (split order—request no egg)
Quantity: 1½ cups
Yosenabe (split order)
Quantity: 1½ cups
Steamed rice
Quantity: 1 cup
Sake
Quantity: 4 oz

Estimated
Nutrient
Evaluation

913 calories
26% calories as fat
24% calories as protein
38% calories as carbohydrate
12% calories as alcohol
106 mg cholesterol
2050 mg sodium (to lower, avoid soup and limit sauce on entrees)

5

Low Sodium Model Meal

Sushi combination
Quantity: 1 order
Tossed salad (request vinegar or lemon wedges)
Quantity: 1–2 cups
Shabu-shabu (use minimal dipping sauce)
Quantity: 1½ cups
Soba noodles
Quantity: 1½ cups

Estimated Nutrient Evaluation

672 calories
25% calories as fat
27% calories as protein
48% calories as carbohydrate
147 mg cholesterol
870 mg sodium

Seasonings, spices, and terms of Japanese cuisine

Bonito–a fish important in Japanese cuisine, a member of the mackeral family; bonito flakes are an important ingredient in the basic stock called dashi.

Daikon–giant white radish; grated daikon is mixed into tempura sauces.

Dashi–an important element in Japanese cooking, dashi is the basic stock made with water, kombu (seaweed), and bonito flakes.

Gyuniku–beef.

Kombu–a Japanese seaweed central to the basic stock, dashi; also used in sauces and as a wrapper for certain dishes.

Mirin–Japanese rice wine, which is used more in sauces than consumed as a beverage; a central ingredient to the sauces and flavors of Japanese cuisine.

Miso–a fermented soy bean paste that comes in various types, thicknesses, and degrees of saltiness; used in soups, sauces, and dressings–a basic ingredient in Japanese cooking.

Nori–a seaweed often toasted prior to using; has a strong flavor and is used to wrap maki sushi.

Sake–fermented rice wine, sake is the national alcoholic beverage of Japan, most often served warm; it is also used as an ingredient in sauces.

Shitake mushrooms–an abundant mushroom in Japanese cookery, it has a woody and fruity flavor; used fresh or dried.

Shoyu–Japanese soy sauce, with light or dark varieties used; it is made from soy beans, wheat, and salt and is an essential ingredient in Japanese cooking.

Teriyaki sauce–sauce used to broil; made from shoyu and mirin, it means "shining broil."

Tofu–soy bean curd, a major source of protein in the Japanese diet; used in soups, salads, and entrees.

Ton–pork.

Tori–chicken.

Vinegar–in Japan, made from rice and lighter and sweeter than the vinegar Americans are used to.

Wakame–a seaweed used for its flavor and texture; available dried.

Wasabi–grated horseradish that is fragrant and less sharp in taste; one of the strongest spices used in Japanese cooking, it is commonly served with raw fish.

10

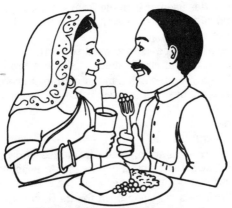

Healthier eating out
Indian Style

Raita or rayta, dahl or dall, nan, and biryani. These are just a sampling of commonly served foods in most Asian Indian restaurants. They don't exactly have the familiar ring of a burger, fries, and Coke. One of the first challenges of learning how to enjoy healthy dining in an Indian restaurant is to acquire the language of Asian Indian cuisine. Beyond the new world of food names, you'll find menu listings spelled differently by one or several letters. It may be vandaloo or vindaloo, samosa or samoosa. The different spellings are due to the phonetic English translations of

Indian languages. The most commonly seen spellings will be used in this chapter, with occasional notations concerning different translations. Recognize that you'll see items spelled differently from restaurant to restaurant.

Being faced with an Indian menu can, to say the least, be quite confusing. To get you up to speed on understanding Indian foods, we'll provide lots of information describing the different menu items typically served and the ingredients used in Indian cooking. In the end, you'll be a pro on picking and choosing the healthiest items an Indian dining spot has to offer. And you'll also understand more about Indian foods and dining practices.

One simply has to look at India's location on a map of the world for clues about the tastes you can expect to find in Indian cuisine. Though Indian food has many unique qualities and cooking techniques, it most closely resembles the cuisine of its neighbors Pakistan, Sri Lanka, Thailand, and Burma. A bit more distant is China, to which there are some, though not as many, similarities. To Americans, Indian food most closely resembles Thai food, both in similarity of spices and ingredients. Curries are commonly served in both countries. They can be quite hot and spicy. Rice is a predominant feature of both cuisines. Basmati rice is the rice of choice in India, and it is frequently used in Indian restaurants in the United States. This long-grained, aromatic rice is unique to India and is considered to be of premium quality.

India is the home of the Himalayan Mountain range and the Indus and Ganges rivers. In India there are quite a multitude of religions. Hinduism, Islam, and Buddhism are three of the most common. Food practices in certain regions of India reflect the predominant religion. For example, vegetarianism is often practiced by Buddhists, and pork and pork products are avoided by Moslems. In fact there appears to be very little pork or pork products used in Indian cooking. Hindus do not eat beef due to their belief in the sanctity of the cow.

Beyond religious mandates, the foods found in different regions of India also vary. Northern Indian food is generally not as hot as Southern cuisine, which makes use of chilies and peppers. The North uses more wheat products, teas, and eggs, whereas the

South features more rice, vegetables, and coffee. There is a greater use of seafood in the areas of southern India that are proximal to the sea. You can expect to find hot pickles and chutneys served in the south. Yogurt is a common ingredient used in both Northern and Southern cookery. It might be said that the Indian food found in American restaurants bends toward Northern regional food practices.

Indian restaurants are growing in numbers and popularity in the United States. This correlates closely with the growing Indian population within our borders. There are presently in the range of a half-million Indians living in the U.S., including first, second, and third generation individuals. There was a small influx of Indians in the early 1900s and the 1960s and 1970s brought a greater number of people who found America a great place for education and personal and professional growth. In the last 20 years there has been a very large influx of Indians from rural India, whereas earlier immigrants came from the cities. Some of these individuals have put their skills to use by becoming restaurateurs. Indians now make their homes in American cities from California to Texas to Massachusetts. Like many newer and less well known ethnic cuisines, it's more common to find Indian restaurants in large urban centers but unlikely to find them in smaller cities and towns.

As is common with many ethnic cuisines, Indian food in America is influenced by the American taste bud and style of eating. Indian restaurants do not seem to distinguish greatly between Southern and Northern-style cuisine. There seem to be many foods that you can simply expect to find listed on most menus, such as the appetizers samosa and pakora and the entrees chicken vindaloo or tandoori. You can also expect to find the accompaniments: mango chutney, dahl, and raita.

If you ate Indian food in a traditional Indian household, you might expect much hotter and spicier tastes. An Indian friend of mine once prepared a chicken biryani dish for a group of us, which I thought was great but on the spicy side. She said that it was very mild compared to how she would prepare it for her family. There has been some "cooling down" of Indian food for the American palate.

Pepper soup, or the more familiar name, mulligatawny, is a regular on the South Indian table. It supposedly aids in digestion. There are a number of different recipes for mulligatawny, from a creamy soup to a very light lentil-based soup. Bombay duck is another example. This is a sauteed or dried white fish served in small pieces with rice and curry dishes. (See "The Spices, Seasonings, and Ingredients of Indian Cuisine" at the end of this chapter.)

Cooking methods frequently used in Indian cuisine are stewing, frying, boiling, and steaming. It's usual to fry appetizers and breads and to have main dishes such as masalas and bhunas stewed. There is a limited amount of food preparation done in the oven. Obviously, some of these cooking techniques have evolved from times when ovens were non-existent. The tandoor, still used today to prepare tandoori chicken and other treats, is a clay oven that uses charcoal.

Typically, the evening meal in an Indian household is eaten between 7:00 and 9:00 P.M. There is a morning meal and an afternoon tea around 4:00–5:00 P.M. The main meal is the evening meal, and it usually consists of a rice dish and a curry dish made either with vegetables, legumes, meat, or seafood. Breads, such as puri or chapati, are always part of the main meal, along with some accompaniments—perhaps raita, dahl, and pickles. Fruits may follow the meal. There is little emphasis on sweet desserts as an important part of the meal.

The way in which food is served for the main meal resembles our concept of family-style service. Small bowls containing the curry dishes, raita, chutneys, and others are placed on the *thali,* a large metal platter. The breads and the small bowls on the thali are put in the middle of a low table, and everyone takes their portion. Each person receives a large individual bowl of rice. Eating with the fingers of the right hand is acceptable, and the bread can be used somewhat like a scoop.

Some Indian restaurants let you order in this family fashion. They list it as "thali" in the vegetable section of the menu. The meal comes with several dishes, rice, choices of bread, raita, and papadum. This might be a good way to order with a group. You get to taste several items in small portions. Be aware of the contents. Make sure, for instance, that you have a choice of bread and can select the much lower fat chapati rather than poori.

It is more common for Indian restaurants to serve American style. You often have the choice of ordering a complete dinner or à la carte. You are better off ordering à la carte as a method of decreasing the quantity of food consumed. As is true in American dining, the soup comes first and appetizers follow. Next the breads, rice, and entree selections are served. Typical of the American style, there is major focus on the entree choice—will it be chicken, beef, or seafood.

Vegetables and legumes play an important role in Indian cooking so it is easy to minimize the protein content of an Indian meal. The tradition of bringing several bowls of condiments as part of the meal is common. You can expect to find hot onion relish or chutney and dahl delivered to your table without requesting it. You might also find mango chutney and raita as well. These accompaniments are typically part of an Indian meal.

Charmaine Solomon, author of *The Complete Asian Cookbook,* defines spices as the "soul" of Indian cooking. What is known as curry, a single spice available in the U.S., is unknown in Indian cooking. Actually, curry translated means "sauce." The main dishes in Indian cooking use a variety of spices to provide the curry flavor.

A garam masala, or fragrant mix of ground spices combined in varying quantities, produces many of the wonderful tastes of Indian cuisine. Some spices frequently found in the garam masala are cardamom, coriander, cumin, cloves, and cinnamon. Several of these spices are referred to as the "fragrant" spices. In the southern regions you might find pepper and chilies added to raise the "heat." Mint, garlic, ginger, yogurt, and coconut milk are other common ingredients in Indian cooking. You'll find more of these spices and ingredients defined in the listing at the end of this chapter.

Another distinctive item present in most Indian meals is basmati rice. As an Indian friend said, once you taste basmati rice, which is a premium rice, you won't want to use any other. Basmati rice is a fragrant, long-grain, white rice. You'll find rice on an Indian menu called pullao or pilau. You can expect it to be basmati rice. Plain pullao is usually served along with the main dish, although peas pullao or pullao with paneer, peas, and nuts is often available. Also basmati rice is the main ingredient in biryani. This is a rice dish that also contains a choice of chicken, beef, shrimp with vegetables, and dried fruits mixed in. It's a good choice because it's low in protein and high in carbohydrates.

What to consider before ordering

As with most ethnic cuisines, there are pros and cons to Indian cookery. If you have some basic knowledge of the cuisine, are careful about reading the food descriptions, and are willing to ask questions as necessary, you will have no problem navigating around an Indian menu. Indian, like many Asian cuisines, can be quite healthy for those interested in keeping fat down, protein low, and pushing those complex, high-fiber carbohydrates.

The pros of Indian food include its accent on carbohydrates and deemphasis of protein. Basmati rice, almost all carbohydrate, is a main element of Indian cuisine. Breads are considered an important part of the meal, although one needs to watch out for the fried varieties. Legumes, including lentils and chick peas, are often found in dishes or accompaniments. These are good sources of soluble fiber and non-animal protein. Remember, soluble fibers are the ones thought to lower blood cholesterol and triglycerides. Vegetables are incorporated into most meals. They might be in curry dishes, biryani, and pullao. Commonly served Indian vegetables are spinach, eggplant, cabbage, potatoes, and peas. Onions, green peppers, and tomatoes are often found in the stewed entrees. Yogurt is frequently used in gravies; it's the plain, low-fat variety.

Another positive aspect that assists in keeping protein, calories, and cholesterol low is the wide availability of chicken and seafood. Beef and lamb are commonly found on the menu but can easily be avoided. Pork and pork products are rarely found on Indian menus. Small quantities of protein are used in each dish. This likely relates back to their minimal availablity. If you share a chicken or shrimp masala, you won't eat much more than two to three ounces of protein each. Also, it's a great idea to order one chicken or seafood dish and one vegetable dish, maybe a biryani or aloo chole. This way you can really keep the protein and cholesterol low.

The negative aspects of Indian cuisine can be the high fat content. Fat finds its way into Indian foods mainly by way of food preparation. Ghee, defined as clarified butter, is a common ingredient. Frying and sauteeing are common preparation methods. For example, most appetizers, such as samosa and pakora, are fried. Many breads are fried, such as paratha and poori.

The initial step in many entree dishes is to saute onions and other ingredients in oil or ghee. The oils most frequently used in Indian cooking are sesame and coconut oil. Sesame is mainly a polyunsaturated oil. However, coconut oil is about the most saturated oil one can use. It is difficult to determine exactly which oil or combination of oils is used in most Indian restaurants in this country. You might want to ask when you are ordering. If the response is coconut oil, it would be best to avoid as much fried food as possible to avoid calories as well as saturated fat.

There is wide use of coconut milk in Indian cooking, and this, too, contributes calories, fat, and saturated fat. Look for the words coconut milk, coconut cream, or simply shredded coconut on the descriptions of menu items and try to avoid these. You might also want to ask which items don't have coconut milk added or if it could be left out.

The sodium content of an Indian meal can be kept within bounds by navigating around the menu carefully. It's best to avoid the soups, which tend to be high in sodium. Many dishes have small amounts of salt added, but if it's divided into a number of servings and you keep the portions small, you'll end up consuming a minimal quantity. Obviously, there are different recipes followed and varying quantities of salt used in cooking.

As many items are prepared to order, try requesting that no salt be added to your dishes. This would be similar to requesting no MSG in Chinese restaurants. And that request seems to be met with ease. Though salt is used in many Indian recipes as a flavor enhancer, the flavor of Indian food certainly does not depend on salt. The other spices used most frequently are sodium-free, so you get lots of taste and next to no sodium. Due to the spiciness and highly seasoned quality of Indian foods, it's unnecessary to use salt after cooking. Actually, it's uncommon to find a salt shaker on the table in an Indian restaurant.

Managing the Menu

Ordering appetizers in an Indian restaurant can present a problem because there are very few that are not deep fried. It's common to find samosas, a turnover stuffed with peas and potatoes and then fried; cheese, chicken, or vegetable pakoras, which are all fried; and fried shrimp with poori. One item that doubles both as an appetizer and a bread is papadum. This is a thin wafer made from spicy lentils. It is fried in its preparation but is quite light and results in the best of the fried choices. If you have some calories to spare, think about just sampling one appetizer. Share one appetizer, which usually comes with two pieces, with your dining partner. If you're with a group and several appetizers or a combination plate (poo poo platter, Indian style) is ordered, decide what's best and take one piece.

Two soups that may be used as openers and nice fillers if you can spare the calories are mulligatawny and lentil soup. They are both seasoned with the common Indian spices. Thus they are quite tasty, consist mainly of carbohydrates, and are relatively low in fat and calories. Creamy soups such as poppy seed and coconut shold be avoided.

Ordering bread from an Indian menu can present some difficulties, but there often are a few more choices than from the appetizer section. Papadum, also seen abbreviated as papad, is the crisp, thin, lentil wafer. Chapati is a flat disc of unleavened bread resembling pita bread; and nan, which is a leavened bread, are all good choices. Poori, a light, puffed fried bread, and paratha, a multi-layered fried bread, should be avoided due to their fat content. Paratha can be stuffed with potatoes or meats, but should also be avoided in this form because it's then fried.

Moving onto the entree selections, you'll find that many of the same preparations are used for chicken, fish, shrimp, beef, and lamb. For instance, you can often get vindaloo prepared with chicken, beef, or fish. There are also potatoes and many common Indian spices added to this particular dish. To keep saturated fat, cholesterol, and calories on the downward side, it's best to stick with fish, chicken, or shrimp. Some dishes using these protein foods are masala, a spice combination with sauteed tomatoes and onions; bhuna, another dish similar to masala; saag, which has spinach and spices added; or a curry dish. Preparations done in a clay oven, or tandoor, are a bit drier and thus lower in fat; tandoori and tikka are often done with chicken. It's best to avoid the malai and korma dishes, which use cream in their preparation.

In most restaurants you'll get plain pullao (basmati rice) as a side dish. Don't make the mistake I did when first eating Indian food of ordering a rice dish, peas pullao, and then having the plain pullao come as well. If you want a special rice dish, ask them not to bring the plain pullao. Biryanis are listed under rice dishes but can be eaten as an entree. They are often made with chicken, lamb, beef, shrimp, or just vegetables. A chicken masala, for instance, could be nicely complemented with a shrimp biryani. That way, you keep the protein and fat content limited.

Vegetable dishes in an Indian restaurant can be used as a main course. From a nutritional standpoint, this is a wise choice. Many vegetable dishes contain a variety of chick peas, lentils, potatoes, spinach, cauliflower, onions, and/or tomatoes. Often they are in curry or cheese sauces. Interestingly, the cheese, or paneer, in Indian food is made from milk and lemon juice, so it actually has much less fat than what we typically think of as cheese.

A unique part of Indian cuisine is the accompaniments, items often listed as condiments. Raita, usually a combination of plain yogurt, cucumber, and onions, though it can have tomatoes or fruit added, is quite healthy. Its purpose is actually to cool the mouth from the hot curry tastes. Dahl is the low-fat, spicy, lentil-based side sauce that is served warm. Onion chutney, sometimes called relish, is a regular accompaniment and often arrives without ordering. It is quite low in calories and adds some zip to the foods. Mango chutney is very popular in U.S. Indian restaurants. It can be quite sweet and contains mainly mango and sugar. Due to the sugar content, it should be used in minimal quantities or not at all by people with diabetes. Other chutneys that are often available are mint and tamarind chutneys.

Salads are often listed, but they do not resemble our idea of a green salad. Ask before ordering so you know what the particular restaurant defines as a salad. Typically, they might be onion or tomato-based. They basically include no dressing other than lemon juice, which is great for the calorie and fat counters. Pickle is another available accompaniment. They are prepared with a variety of low-calorie ingredients and hot spices. All accompaniments are served and eaten in very small quantities.

Desserts are typically deemphasized in India and can remain that way when you eat Indian cuisine in America. You might find koulfi, which is a rich ice cream with nuts, or several custards and puddings, kheers. Obviously, it's best if desserts are avoided. They generally will simply provide more calories and fat. If you must, use the portion control strategy of sharing—one dessert, several forks or spoons, whichever is most appropriate.

A variety of the usual low to no-calorie beverages are found in Indian restaurants. Low-calorie soda, water, coffee, and tea are almost always available. Darjeeling, an Indian tea, is usually listed and is nice to try for a different taste. There are several sweetened Indian drinks to avoid, such as a lassi, a sweetened yogurt drink. There are several Indian beers that you might find listed; however, they are not often light beer. Singha beer, which is actually a Thai beer, is often served at Indian restaurants. But King Fisher is an authentic Indian beer and also regularly available.

As you can see, there should be no problem choosing a healthy meal in an Indian restaurant. Simply watch out for the fats, fried foods, and overeating. Most Indian restaurant menus do provide at least a brief description of all items. If you don't have enough information, don't be embarrassed to ask questions. You want to feel comfortable and enjoy what you've ordered. Limiting portions is not too difficult because the size of most dishes tends to be small. Watch out for over-ordering and, remember, you will get several condiments and basmati rice without even saying "I'll have. . . ."

When the menu arrives, look for certain key words and phrases that signal the nutritional advisability of the items. We call them "Green Flag" (go for it) and "Red Flag" (steer clear) words.

Green Flag Words

tikka (pan roasted)
cooked with or marinated in
  yogurt
cooked with green vegetables
cooked with onions, tomatoes, peppers, and/or mushrooms
with spinach (saag)
baked leavened bread
masala
tandoori
paneer*
cooked with curry
marinated in spices
cooked in hot spices
lentils
garnished with dried fruits
chick peas and potatoes
basmati rice (pullao)
matta (peas)
kebab

Red Flag Words

fritters
fried
dipped in batter
dipped in chick pea batter
deep fried
korma
stuffed and fried
creamy curry sauce
ghee*
butter, made with butter
garnished with nuts
almonds, pistachios
rich cream sauce
cooked in cream sauce
creamy tomato sauce
molee (coconut)
coconut milk or soup

*Words defined in "The Spices,
  Seasonings, and Ingredients of
  Indian Cuisine," following.

**Special
Requests
Indian
Style**

Please bring the accompaniments raita, dahl, and onion chutney.

If a special rice is ordered, request that the plain pullao not be brought.

My order will be à la carte, not a complete dinner.

Please don't garnish with nuts.

Please don't garnish with dried fruits.

Is it possible to prepare my dish without adding any salt?

Please don't use extra salt in the preparation.

Please bring my soup when you bring the appetizers for the others.

Please bring my salad when the others have their appetizers.

I'll have a cup of Darjeeling tea with my meal.

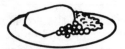

Typical Menu: Indian Style

Appetizers   **Cheese pakoras** (homemade cheese deep-fried in chick pea batter)
✓**Samosa** (vegetable turnover, stuffed and fried)
Fried shrimp with poori (shrimp with onions and peppers fried with spices)
✓**Papadum** (also seen as papad) (crispy, thin lentil wafers)
Chicken pakoras (chunks of boneless chicken marinated in spicy sauce, then fried)
Shami kebab (ground meat patty, fried)

Soups   ✓**Mulligatawny** (lentil, vegetables, and spices)
Coconut soup (coconut cream and pistachio nuts)
Poppy seed soup (almond, poppy seed, milk, and coconut cream)
✓**Dahl rasam** (pepper soup with lentils)

Breads (Roti)   **Paratha** (shallow-fried multi-layered bread made with butter)
Poori (light, puffed fried bread)
✓**Chapati** (thin, dry whole-wheat bread)
Aloo paraha (paratha stuffed with potatoes, made with butter
✓**Nan** (leavened baked bread topped with poppy seeds)
✓**Kulcha** (leavened baked bread)

✓*Preferred Choice*

Chicken (Murgi)	✓**Chicken tandoori** (marinated in spices and roasted in a tandoor, or clay oven)
	✓**Chicken tikka** (roasted in charcoal oven with mild spices)
	✓**Chicken saag** (boneless chicken cooked with spinach)
	✓**Chicken vandaloo** (boneless chicken cooked with potatoes and hot spices)
	Chicken kandhari (chicken cooked with cream sauce and cashews)
	✓**Chicken masala** (roasted chicken cooked in spices and thick curry sauce)
Shrimp/ Fish	**Shrimp malai** (cooked with cream, mushrooms, and coconut)
	✓**Shrimp bhuna** (cooked with green vegetables, onions, and tomatoes)
	✓**Fish masala** (boneless fish marinated in a spicy yogurt sauce)
	Shrimp curry (cooked in a thick curry sauce)
	✓**Fish vandaloo** (boneless fish cooked with potatoes and hot spices)
Beef/Lamb	✓**Lamb bhuna** (pan roasted with spices, onions, and tomatoes)
	✓**Lamb saag** (cooked with spinach in a spicy curry sauce)
	✓**Beef vandaloo** (beef curry cooked with potatoes and hot spices)
	✓**Kheema matter** (minced lamb and peas cooked with fresh herbs)
	Beef korma (beef curry cooked with cream)
Rice (Pullao)	✓**Shrimp biryani** (shrimp cooked with basmati rice and garnished with dried fruits)
	✓**Vegetable biryani** (basmati rice cooked with green vegetables and garnished with dried fruits)

✓**Plain pullao** (basmati rice cooked with saffron)

✓**Peas pullao** (basmati rice cooked with peas)

✓**Shrimp pullao** (shrimp cooked with basmati rice)

Vegetables ✓**Vegetable curry** (green peas, tomatoes, and cauliflower)

Vegetable korma (mixed vegetables cooked with cream, herbs, and cashews)

✓**Saag paneer** (spinach cooked with homemade cheese)

✓**Matter paneer** (homemade cheese and green peas curry)

✓**Aloo chole** (chick peas cooked with tomatoes and potatoes)

Accompaniments ✓**Raita** (rayta) (yogurt with grated cucumbers, onions, and spices)

✓**Mango chutney**

Mint chutney

✓**Onion chutney** (diced onions with hot spices)

Tamarind sauce

Dahl (lentil sauce)

✓**Tamata salat** (diced tomatoes and onions with hot spices and lemon)

Desserts **Koulfi** (rich ice cream with almonds and pistachios)

Mango koulfi

Gulab jamun (fried milk balls soaked in sugar syrup, served warm)

Ras malai (homemade cheese in sweetened milk)

Now that you've seen what may be available on the menu, look over the following five "Model Meals" for suggestions on how to order to achieve specific nutritional goals. Models are numbered one to five for quick reference, and each is followed by an "Estimated Nutrient Evaluation" that analyzes the content of that meal.

May I Take Your Order

Healthy	30% Calories as fat
Daily	20% Calories as protein
Eating	50% Calories as carbohydrate
Goals	300 mg/day Cholesterol
	3000 mg/day Sodium

Low Calorie/
Low Fat
Model Meal

Nan
Quantity: ¼ loaf
Exchanges: 1 fat; 1 starch
Shrimp biryani
Quantity: 1½ cups
Exchanges: 2 meat; 1 fat; 1
   vegetable; 2 starch
Raita
Quantity: 3 tbsp
Exchanges: ½ vegetable
Onion chutney
Quantity: 2 tbsp
Exchanges: ½ vegetable
Tamata salat
Quantity: ½ cup
Exchanges: 1 vegetable
Darjeeling tea
Quantity: 2 cups
Exchanges: free

Estimated
Nutrient
Evaluation

480 calories
25% calories as fat
24% calories as protein
50% calories as carbohydrate
128 mg cholesterol
950 mg sodium

2

Low Calorie/ Low Cholesterol Model Meal	**Dahl rasam soup** *Quantity:* 1 cup **Fish masala** *Quantity:* 1½ cups **Plain pullao** *Quantity:* 1 cup **Raita** *Quantity:* 3 tbsp **Mango chutney** *Quantity:* 2 tbsp **Pickle** *Quantity:* 1 tbsp

Estimated Nutrient Evaluation	540 calories 23% calories as fat 22% calories as protein 55% calories as carbohydrate 60 mg cholesterol 1400 mg sodium

 3

Higher Calorie/Low Fat Model Meal	**Samosa** *Quantity:* 1 piece *Exchanges:* 2 fat; 1 starch **Chicken tandoori** *Quantity:* 4 oz (split order) *Exchanges:* 4 meat (lean); 1 fat **Peas pullao** *Quantity:* 1½ cups *Exchanges:* 3 starch **Saag paneer** *Quantity:* 1 cup *Exchanges:* 1 fat; 2 vegetable; ½ milk **Mint Chutney** *Quantity:* 2 tbsp *Exchanges:* free **Dahl** *Quantity:* 3 tbsp *Exchanges:* ½ starch

Estimated Nutrient Evaluation	852 calories
	38% calories as fat
	23% calories as protein
	39% calories as carbohydrate
	93 mg cholesterol
	1700 mg sodium

❹
Higher Calorie/Low Cholesterol Model Meal

Papadum
Quantity: 1 slice
Lamb Bhuna
Quantity: 1½ cups
Plain pullao
Quantity: 1 cup
Vegetable curry
Quantity: 1 cup
Tamata salat
Quantity: ½ cup
Mango chutney
Quantity: 3 tbsp
White wine
Quantity: 6 oz

Estimated Nutrient Evaluation	949 calories
	31% calories as fat
	17% calories as protein
	39% calories as carbohydrate
	13% calories as alcohol
	102 mg cholesterol
	1200 mg sodium

❺
Low Sodium Model Meal

Samosa
Quantity: 1 piece
Chicken tikka
Quantity: 4 oz
Plain pullao
Quantity: 1 cup
Aloo chole
Quantity: ¾ cup

> **Raita**
> *Quantity:* 3 tbsp
> **Mango chutney**
> *Quantity:* 3 tbsp
> **Singha beer**
> *Quantity:* 12 oz

Estimated Nutrient Evaluation	
	890 calories
	32% calories as fat
	19% calories as protein
	38% calories as carbohydrate
	11% calories as alcohol
	80 mg cholesterol
	900 mg sodium

The spices, seasonings, and ingredients of Indian cuisine

Bombay duck–this term does not describe a bird but rather fish served either sauteed, fried, or dried, along with curries and rice; not often seen on U.S. Indian menus.

Cardamom–expensive spice native to India, in the ginger family. Either the whole cardamom pod or only seeds are used; one of the most common spices found in garam masalas (curry mixtures).

Cinnamon–delicate spice commonly found in spice combinations used in curries and rarely as the ground spice typically used in the U.S.; stick cinnamon with more intense flavor is used in India.

Clove–another commonly used spice in curries, it is the dried flower bud of an evergreen tropical tree found in Southeast Asia.

Coconut milk–not the liquid found inside the coconut, it is a creamy fluid extracted from the flesh of the coconut.

Coriander–fragrant spice often the main ingredient in curries; either ground coriander or the whole leaf is used. Also called cilantro or Chinese parsley.

Cumin–another fragrant spice important to curry dishes; used as either seeds or ground.

Curry–as an individual spice, "curry" is not used in Indian cooking. The word means "sauce," and many spices, individually roasted, make up the curry mixture, known as garam masala.

Fennel–another spice used in curries; a member of the cumin family and on occasion referred to as sweet cumin.

Ghee–clarified butter; contains none of the milk solids.

Malai–a thick cream made by separating and collecting the top part of boiled milk; used in entrees for a thick, creamy sauce.

Mint–used to add flavor to curry dishes and also as a main ingredient in mint chutney and mint sambal; used in biryani and as a dipping sauce for appetizers.

Paneer–referred to as homemade cream or cottage cheese and made from milk curdled with lemon juice and strained through cheese cloth. Paneer is used in vegetable and rice dishes. For vegetarians, it is a complete protein source.

Poppy seeds– ground to a powder and used in curry dishes to thicken the gravies.

Rose water–flavoring agent used in Indian desserts; extracted from rose petals by steaming and then diluting the essence.

Saffron–known as the most expensive spice in the world, small quantities are used commonly in Indian cooking. Obtained by drying the stamens of saffron crocus, saffron strands are thread-like and deep orange in color.

Tamarind–used for its acidic quality, it is a fruit from a large tropical tree; a commonly used Indian spice or food.

Tumeric–spice which lends the yellow-orange color to commercial curry. Part of the ginger family and commonly used in Indian cooking.

Yogurt–called *dahl* in India, a common ingredient in Indian cooking; always plain and unflavored.

11

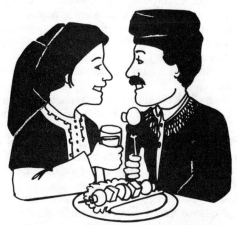

Healthier eating out
Middle Eastern Style

Pita bread, hummus, baba ghanoush, tabooli, and kalamata (olives) are quickly becoming familiar foods in American supermarkets. Though they might be foreign to many people, they're regulars on most Middle Eastern, Armenian, Israeli, and Greek restaurant menus. Middle Eastern restaurants are not as plentiful, especially in the heartland of America, as Italian or Chinese dining spots, but the number is on the rise. Over the last century, more Middle Easterners have emigrated to the U.S., and, as usual, this pattern has resulted in more Middle Eastern restaurants. It has also created a demand to have Middle Eastern foods available on supermarket shelves. These foods present Americans with another interesting and healthy cuisine to join our already diverse repertory.

It's important initially to define what is meant by "Middle Eastern cuisine." There are strong similarities among the foods native to Greece, Syria, Lebanon, Iran, Iraq, Turkey, Armenia (now part of the Soviet Union), and Israel. There are also commonalities among Middle Eastern foods and those indigenous to North Africa, the countries of Morocco, Egypt, Tunisia, Algeria, and Libya. Certainly, there are individualities, but there's more in common than unique, especially when viewing the region from a global perspective.

You'll see differences in the spellings of foods from menu to menu and cookbook to cookbook. For instance, hummus, as it is most commonly written, is also spelled "homos," "hummos," and "hoomis." Some of the different spellings might also be due to the English transliteration. Pronunciation of words can also vary tremendously. It might simply be that the accent falls on different parts of the word or spelling varies.

A brief look into the history of the Middle East, perhaps one of the oldest civilized areas of the world, reveals some reasons why the foods are so similar. As Claudia Roden writes in *A Book of Middle Eastern Food,* "the history of this food is that of the Middle East." There were times when Greeks and Romans ruled this area. More recent history finds the Middle East long dominated by Turkish rule. And early in the nineteenth century France and Britain had their stint at controlling parts of the Middle East. Today, most of these countries are independent.

The Middle East has been, and continues to be, a hotbed of political unrest. The search for political stability, education, and economic opportunity are the most frequent reasons for emigration. Two waves of emigration from the Middle East occurred. The first was from the late 1800s to the early 1900s, and the second took place after World War II. Immigration of Middle Easterners continues today. It is not uncommon to find new immigrants seeking economic independence in the food or restaurant business. The obvious result is an increased number of restaurants.

Middle Eastern restaurants in America

Whether the food is delineated as Greek, Israeli, Armenian, Moroccan, or just plain Middle Eastern, these foods are found at a broad spectrum of restaurants. You'll find Middle Eastern restaurants, simple or more upscale, that are solely dedicated to serving the traditional foods. So items such as baba ghanoush, lamb shish kebabs, kibbeh, and the very sweet dessert baklava almost always appear on the menu.

Middle Eastern foods are also represented in mall eateries. You'll find spots serving gyros or souvlaki wrapped in pita bread with lettuce, tomatoes, onions, and topped with tzateki sauce. Or you might see fast food stops serving the Middle Eastern regulars, falafel, fattoush salad, or tabooli. Some foods have become integrated into the items served at "American" restaurants. You find sandwiches available on pita bread, feta cheese is sprinkled on a salad, or rice pilaf is served as a side dish. Today, it's quite common to see a so-called Greek salad or gyros wrapped in pita bread on the menu at Italian or American lunch spots. These are usually lunch spots that also serve pizza, submarine sandwiches, and antipastos.

Foods of the Middle East

As usual, the foods that play a predominant role in Middle Eastern cooking are foods that are naturally plentiful in that region. Wheat, grains, legumes, olives, dates, figs, lamb, and eggplant are just a few of the ingredients central to Middle Eastern cooking.

Rice, combined with a variety of ingredients into rice pilaf, is commonly served in Greece and the Middle East, whereas couscous, made with cracked wheat, is more indigenous to North African countries. Tabooli, the cold cracked wheat or bulghur salad marinated with raw vegetables, is most familiar in Lebanon, though served throughout the Middle East.

Pita pockets, as they are often called in America, are well integrated into American culture. Pita is a flat, round bread only slightly leavened. Due to the very hot oven in which it is cooked, steam is created and the process results in a hollow center. This "pocket" makes it perfect for stuffing. Another health benefit of pita bread is that it is low in fat and therefore calories. As Ken Haedrich explains in his article "Pita Principles" in the *Country Journal*, "Once almost unheard of in this country outside of Middle Eastern enclaves, pita has emerged in the eighties as the repository for almost anything edible, from burgers, sprouts, and salads to more traditional fillings like hummus, tabouli, and kibbeh."

It's common to find stuffed dishes. Probably the best known are dolma, stuffed grape leaves. There are also stuffed cabbage and stuffed eggplant. They all can be stuffed with meat or meatless mixtures.

Chick peas, fava beans, and other legumes are indigenous to the Middle East. Chick peas and fava beans are pureed together to make falafel or ta'amia. Chick peas are mashed and mixed with tahini (sesame seed paste, or puree) to make the familiar hummus.

Due to the plentifulness of olives, olive oil is frequently the product of choice. It is more predominantly used in cold dishes. Olives, both green and black, are frequently served. It is a rare Greek salad that doesn't have at least two or more Greek olives. These very salty olives, which are soaked in brine, are called kalamata.

One sees limited use of seafood in Middle Eastern cookery. Other than legumes and grains, lamb is the most familiar protein food. Beef is also used but to a lesser degree. Eggs are used quite a bit, especially in soups such as avgolemono, egg and lemon sauce, and also in some of the pasta dishes or spinach and cheese pies.

Milk is not frequently drunk in the Middle East due in part to the high incidence of lactose intolerance. Yogurt is frequently used, served plain as a side dish or mixed with garlic, mint, and salt. Yogurt might be found as a dressing for salads, in soups, or as a base in sauces such as tzateki. The purpose of yogurt, as in Indian cuisine, is to act as a refresher, or soother from the spiciness. Two cheeses, feta and kasseri, are commonly used in Middle Eastern cookery, served alone or incorporated into appetizers, salads, and entrees.

Phyllo (also filo or fila), which literally means leaf, is the paper thin Middle Eastern dough. It's used to make sweet desserts, such as baklava, or dinner pies, such as spanikopita, the well-known spinach and feta cheese pie. The dough itself is made from flour, egg, water, and some oil or butter. When phyllo dough is

used, the layers are separated and liberally coated
with butter. Obviously this technique quickly raises
calories.

Another historical trait common to Middle Eastern
cooking is that from very few ingredients many different dishes are created. Similar vegetables, such as
eggplant, onions, and tomatoes, are found in raw
vegetable salads, in meatless casseroles, with ground
lamb, and stuffed into grape leaves.

The geographic locale also has an impact on ingredients, spices, and flavors of the foods served. Commonly used spices are parsley, mint, cilantro, and
oregano. Others include spices that are also mainstays
in Indian cooking—cumin, coriander, cinnamon, and
ginger. Long ago, the Middle East was a major link
on the spice route between the Far East and Europe
and from Europe to Africa.

Food preparation and service

Cooking methods currently used reflect those passed
down through the generations. They reflect the ab-
sence of modern conveniences such as ranges and
refrigerators. It's common to see foods grilled, such
as shish kebab; fried, as is falafel; ground, as is kibbeh; or stewed, as with couscous. Marinating is a favorite preparation method for vegetables and meats.
Pickled vegetables are served, originally a method of
food preservation. Basically, the cooking methods are
simple.

The main meal in typical Middle Eastern style is
eaten at midday. It consists of a meat stew or meatballs and a stuffed item, which might contain mixtures of vegetables, ground beef and/or lamb, and
legumes. In addition there is always a grain, perhaps
rice pilaf, couscous, or tabooli, depending on the country; bread, often pita; a salad or raw vegetable combination; and yogurt as a side dish. The meal is
usually concluded simply with a bowl of fresh fruit
set on the table. The sweets or pastries are served
several hours after the meal, with the familiar strong
Greek or Turkish coffee. Baklava, kataif, and rice pudding are common Middle Eastern desserts.

Middle Eastern restaurants, quick eating spots, and
upscale establishments seem to offer a truer rendi-
tion of the foods from their homeland than do other
ethnic cuisines. So if you have visited the Middle East,

you are likely to see very similar foods and preparation methods used in America, whereas this is not as true for Chinese or Mexican cuisine.

What to consider before ordering

In general, Middle Eastern foods are a good match with healthy eating goals. There are many vegetables, both raw in spicy salads and cooked in tomato-based sauces. Legumes are widely used and due to their soluble fiber content, they assist in lowering blood cholesterol. The higher fat red meats are used more than chicken and fish, but the saving grace is that quantities are limited. The meat is often mixed with vegetables and/or grains, and you are not served large portions of meat, as is common practice in American cuisine. As usual, fats, from a variety of sources, will raise calories quicker than anything. Basically, it's easy to keep the carbos up and the protein and fat down if you pick your Middle Eastern menu offerings wisely.

Fats, of course, are your enemy. It's important to recognize all the ways in which fat can creep into Middle Eastern foods and keep an eye out for these when perusing the menu. As discussed, olives, rich in fat, are indigenous to the Middle East, and therefore olives and their byproducts show up in appetizers, salad dressings, marinades, and entrees. The oils used for deep frying are likely to be corn or nut oils. Obviously, it's important to avoid fried foods, such as falafel. Eggplant dishes can be high in fat simply because eggplant absorbs huge quantities of oil, and it's often fried before being incorporated into a casserole. But it's actually easy to avoid fried foods on a Middle Eastern menu because there are many other healthy choices.

Butter is traditionally used in several items, such as spinach and cheese pies, and most foods made with phyllo dough, such as baklava or kataif. Fat also creeps in by way of seeds and nuts commonly used in cooking. Tahini, ground sesame seed paste, is basically all fat. Granted it's mainly polyunsaturated. Tahini is used in hummus and baba ghanoush and might turn up in salad dressings and sauces. Pine nuts are found in some casserole dishes; walnuts are used in desserts.

Eggs are frequently found in Middle eastern cooking, either in appetizers, soups, spinach pie, omelettes, or thick sauces. It's best to avoid the obvious sources of eggs if you're closely monitoring cholesterol.

The sodium content of a Middle Eastern meal doesn't need to skyrocket, especially if you are aware of the real danger foods. Several Middle Eastern regulars are quite high in sodium—feta and kasseri cheese, kalamata (olives), and lokaniko (sausage). Salt is consistently used in Middle Eastern food preparation, but not in huge quantities. In addition, many of the flavorings and spices used are very low in sodium—garlic, lemon, dill, parsley, mint, onion, and yogurt.

Managing the menu

The appetizers, or mezze, as they are referred to in the Middle East, are traditionally eaten very leisurely. There are several items you'll find listed both as appetizers and entrees, such as dolma, falafel, and spanikopita. Several of the appetizers are high in fat and best avoided: spanikopita, falafel, taramosalata, and cheese casserole. The frequently offered baba ghanoush and hummus contain tahini, which boosts the fat; they are often served with pita bread, and small quantities are fine.

The best way to keep fat and calories down is to pass right over to the salad. There are multiple salad offerings on a Middle Eastern menu. Greek or house salad is usually lettuce-based with cucumbers, tomatoes, onion, and likely the high-sodium ingredients of feta cheese and olives added. You can certainly ask for dressing on the side. You might find fattoush on the menu, which is a common Middle Eastern salad. It contains cucumbers, tomatoes, onions, and chips of toasted pita bread. This salad might already be dressed prior to serving. Tabouli, the cracked wheat mixture, and tomato and cucumber salad are also regulars and very healthy.

The spices and seasoning frequently used on salads are light and keep the calories down compared to our calorie-laden dressings. Olive oil, lemon or vinegar, mint, parsley, garlic, and salt and pepper are the usual ingredients.

The soup entries are minimal on Middle Eastern menus. Lemon-egg soup, avgolemono, seems to be a regular offering but one to be avoided due to the egg content. There might be a healthy lentil, vegetable, or yogurt-based soup on the menu, all of which are quite healthy.

Middle Eastern entrees are often combination dishes. They contain meat and cracked wheat, with vegetables and spices added, such as kibbeh; or it might be kafta, which is ground beef with onions, parsley, and spices. If desired, it's easy enough to stay vegetarian when eating Middle Eastern food by eating a stuffed eggplant dish, meatless dolma, or just ordering à la carte.

Grilling, stove-top cooking, and baking are used to prepare most dishes. One of the most familiar entrees is shish kebab. Its origins relate back to when the Ottoman armies had to camp outdoors and cook quickly. They devised this method of skewering vegetables and meats together. In most restaurants shish kebab is available with lamb, beef, chicken, and occasionally shrimp. Sometimes a combination is available. The meats are typically marinated in olive oil, lemon, wine, and spices, then grilled on a skewer with vegetables.

Eggplant is seen in several dishes; mousaka is one of the more familiar offerings, or you might find stuffed eggplant with meat, Sheikh el Mahshi. It's important to realize that eggplant can absorb lots of oils and that often, prior to cooking, eggplant has been salted to remove the bitter taste. Mousaka, due to its high fat content, is best avoided.

Gyros meat, a spicy combination of lamb and beef, and souvlaki, which is lamb, are often available wrapped in pitas or served on platters. Both also come with lettuce, tomato, onion, and a spicy yogurt-based sauce called tzateki. Both are fine choices; however, be careful to eat more bread and go light on the meat.

Lah me june is the Armenian answer to the Italian pizza. It is defined as Armenian style pizza, topped with ground meat, parsley, tomatoes, onions, and Middle Eastern spices. This is a good choice because it's low on the protein and high in carbos.

Omelets, made with feta cheese or lokaniko (sausage) and three eggs, are offered on Middle Eastern menus. These are best avoided. Adding cheese or sausage to three eggs is adding insult to injury, and on top of that fat is used in the preparation.

Dinners in Middle Eastern restaurants are usually served with a small salad, pita bread, rice pilaf, and/or a steamed vegetable. All of these offer some safe, relatively low-fat additions to your meal. If you are closely watching your calories, you might need to pick and choose; obviously, the salad and pita bread are good selections. When ordering, don't feel that you must order a dinner. That may simply be too much food. Try ordering à la carte—think about an appetizer of baba ghanoush, dolma stuffed with lamb and rice, and tabooli salad. The appetizer portions are smaller and will allow you to taste more offerings. The same mission can be accomplished by sharing several different items, from appetizers to desserts. Just order one dinner for two, try a couple of low-fat appetizers, and then if it fits into your meal plan, there's room to split a dessert.

Dessert is traditionally just a bowl of fruit, but in most Middle Eastern restaurants in America you'll see the desserts baklava, kataif, and rice pudding listed. Anyone who has had baklava knows that it is probably one of the richest desserts known to humankind. Baklava is made with phyllo dough, plenty of butter, nuts, sugar, and spices. A half-piece is often enough to quench your sweet tooth for quite a while. The other half of enjoying pastries in the Middle East is drinking a cup of very strong Turkish coffee. Depending on the restaurant, it might be called Israeli, Greek, or Turkish coffee, but it all resembles espresso in that it is very strong and served in a demitasse. The coffee alone might be a new taste treat to enjoy, and best yet, it essentially has no calories if it is unsweetened.

When the menu arrives, look for certain key words and phrases that signal the nutritional advisability of the items. We call them "Green Flag" (go for it) and "Red Flag" (steer clear) words.

Green Flag Words

lemon dressing, lemon juice
blended or seasoned with Middle Eastern spices
herbs, herbs and spices
mashed chick peas
fava beans
smoked eggplant
with tomatoes, onions, green peppers, and/or cucumbers
spiced ground meat

special garlic sauce
basted with tomato sauce
garlic
chopped parsley and/or onion
cracked wheat
grape vines or leaves
stuffed with ground lamb or meat
stuffed with rice and imported
  spices
grilled on a skewer
marinated and barbecued
baked
charbroiled or charcoal broiled
stewed or simmered

**Red Flag
Words**

caviar+
tahini
sesame paste or puree
olive oil, pure olive oil
eggs
kalamata olives*
feta cheese*
kasseri cheese
lokaniko*
tarator sauce
lemon and butter sauce
cheese pie
topped with creamy sauce
béchamel sauce
in pastry crust
phyllo dough
pan fried
golden fried

*high in sodium in addition to fat
+high in sodium and cholesterol

**Special
Requests
Middle
Eastern
Style**

Please bring the dressing for my salad on the side.

Please serve the tzateki (or other sauces) on the side.

I'll have the appetizer portion, but I would like that served when you serve the others their entrees.

We're simply going to have salad and share a few appetizers.

Can you leave the feta cheese and olives off the salad; I'm watching my sodium consumption?

Please bring my salad when you bring the appetizers for the others.

Please bring an extra plate because we're going to do some sharing.

Could you bring my cup of soup when the others are having appetizers?

Could I get a doggie bag when you bring the entrees because I'd like to put half away for tomorrow?

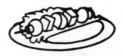

Typical Menu: Middle Eastern Style

Appetizers ✓**Hummus bi tahini** with pita
bread (mashed chick peas blended
with tahini, lemon juice, and
spices)

✓**Baba ghanoush** with pita bread
(smoked eggplant mashed and
combined with tahini, lemon juice,
garlic, and other spices)

Taramosalata with pita bread
(caviar blended with lemon juice
and olive oil)

Kasseri casserole (kasseri cheese
fried with a lemon and butter
sauce)

Spanikopita (spinach and feta
cheese pie made with phyllo
dough)

✓**Dolma** (cold grape leaves stuffed
with a spicy combination of rice,
onions, and tomatoes)

✓**Dolma** (hot grape leaves stuffed
with a spicy combination of
ground lamb, rice, and onions)

Falafel (blend of chick peas and
fava beans, fried and served with
tarator or tahini)

✓**Ful Medames** (fava beans and
chick peas blended with spices
and seasonings)

✓**Cold combination** (tabooli,
hummus bi tahini, and baba
ghanoush)

Hot combination (falafel,
spanikopita, and dolma)

✓*Preferred Choice*

Salads   ✓**Greek salad** (lettuce, tomato, cucumbers, onions, feta cheese, and olives, served with a spicy light lemon and olive oil dressing)
✓**Middle Eastern salad** (lettuce, onions, cucumbers, tomato, mint, parsley, and spices, served with a spicy olive oil and vinegar dressing)
✓**Tabooli** (cracked wheat combined with parsley, tomatoes, cucumbers, lemon, and a spicy dressing)
✓**Fattoush** (lettuce, peppers, scallions, onions, tomatoes, and pieces of toasted pita bread, tossed and served with a light garlic and lemon dressing)
✓**Tomato and cucumber salad** (diced cucumbers and tomatoes marinated in a spicy, light dressing)

Soups   **Avgolemono** (chicken-broth-based soup with eggs and lemon)
✓**Lentil soup** (lentils simmered with zucchini, celery, onions, potatoes, and Middle Eastern spices)

Entrees*   ✓**Shish kebab** (chunks of beef, lamb, or chicken marinated and spiced, skewered with tomatoes, onions, and peppers and grilled)
Mousaka (layers of eggplant, ground lamb, and cheese topped with béchamel sauce)
Spanikopita (spinach and cheese pie made with phyllo dough)
✓**Kibbeh,** baked (cracked wheat mixed with spicy ground meat and stuffed with sauteed onions and pine nuts)

✓**Gyros,** available in a pita or on platter (combination of seared, spicy lamb and beef, served with lettuce, tomato, onions, and tzateki sauce)

✓**Sheik el Mahshi** (baked eggplant, stuffed with ground lamb, pine nuts, onions, Middle Eastern spices, and tomato sauce)

✓**Souvlaki,** available in pita or on platter (marinated and grilled meat, served with lettuce, tomato, onions, and tzateki sauce)

Pasticchio (baked macaroni with ground beef and eggs, topped with a creamy sauce)

Fried kalamaria (squid)

✓**Dolma** (stuffed grape leaves, with ground lamb, rice, onions, and spices)

Falafel (fava beans and chick peas blended with spices and served with tahini or tarator sauce)

✓**Lah me june** (Armenian pizza, topped with ground meat, parsley, tomatoes, onions, and spices)

✓**Kafta** (beef ground with parsley, onions, and other spices and served grilled)

✓**Couscous** (a wheat grain steamed on top of a spicy lamb and vegetable stew)

Omelets (three eggs combined with choice of feta cheese, lokaniko, chicken livers, or any combination)

*Each entree is served with a choice of Middle Eastern salad or steamed vegetable and rice pilaf

Side	✓**Tabooli**
Dishes	✓**Rice pilaf** (long-grain rice sea-soned with butter and saffron)
	✓**Steamed vegetable** combination
	Feta cheese
	Kalamata (olives)
	✓**Pita bread**
Desserts	**Baklava** (pastry made with layers of phyllo dough, nuts, and sugar)
	Kataif (pastry made with shred-ded dough, nuts, and sugar)
	Rice pudding
	Assorted Middle Eastern pastries
	✓**Turkish coffee**
	✓**American coffee**

Now that you've seen what may be available on the menu, look over the following five "Model Meals" for suggestions on how to order to achieve specific nutritional goals. Models are numbered one to five for quick reference, and each is followed by an "Estimated Nutrient Evaluation" that analyzes the content of that meal.

May I Take Your Order

Healthy	30% Calories as fat
Daily	20% Calories as protein
Eating	50% Calories as carbohydrate
Goals	300 mg/day Cholesterol
	3000 mg/day Sodium

❶

Low Calorie/	**Tabooli salad**
Low Fat	*Quantity:* ¾ cup
Model Meal	*Exchanges:* 1 fat; ½ vegetable; 1 starch
	Gyros plate or platter
	Quantity: 3 oz
	Exchanges: 3 meat (med.); 1 vegetable
	Pita bread
	Quantity: ¾ pita
	Exchanges: 2 starch
	Low-calorie carbonated beverage
	Quantity: unlimited
	Exchanges: free

Estimated	560 calories
Nutrient	32% calories as fat
Evaluation	26% calories as protein
	42% calories as carbohydrate
	75 mg cholesterol
	1000 mg sodium

❷

Low Calorie/	**Dolma** cold, without meat (split order)
Low	*Quantity:* 3
Cholesterol	**Greek salad** (dressing on the side)
Model Meal	*Quantity:* 1–2 cups
	Dressing (request extra lemon wedges)
	Quantity: 1 tbsp

Lah me june (Armenian pizza)
Quantity: 8-in. round
Turkish coffee
Quantity: unlimited

Estimated Nutrient Evaluation	612 calories 35% calories as fat 22% calories as protein 43% calories as carbohydrate 75 mg cholesterol 1120 mg sodium

❸
Higher Calorie/Low Fat Model Meal

Fattoush (dressing on the side)
Quantity: 1–2 cups
Exchanges: 2 vegetable; ½ starch
Dressing (on the side)
Quantity: 1 tbsp
Exchanges: 1 fat
Sheik el Mahshi (split order)
Quantity: 1½ cups
Exchanges: 1 meat (med.); 1 fat; 2 vegetables
Kibbeh, baked (split order)
Quantity: 1 cup
Exchanges: 1 meat (med.); 1 vegetable; 1 starch
Rice pilaf
Quantity: ⅔ cup
Exchanges: 1 fat; 2 starch
Retsina wine
Quantity: 6 oz
Exchanges: account for calories but don't omit exchanges

Estimated Nutrient Evaluation	826 calories 33% calories as fat 15% calories as protein 38% calories as carbohydrate 14% calories as alcohol 50 mg cholesterol 1110 mg sodium

❹
**Higher
Calorie/Low
Cholesterol
Model Meal**

Hummus bi tahini
Quantity: ⅓ cup
Pita bread
Quantity: ½ pita
Tomato and cucumber salad
Quantity: ½ cup
Rice pilaf
Quantity: 1 cup
Shish kebab (combination lamb
  and chicken)
Quantity: 2 skewers (about 4 oz
  meat)
Light beer
Quantity: 12 oz

**Estimated
Nutrient
Evaluation**

866 calories
28% calories as fat
20% calories as protein
43% calories as carbohydrate
 9% calories as alcohol
100 mg cholesterol
1260 mg sodium

❺
**Low Sodium
Model Meal**

Baba ghanoush
Quantity: ½ cup
Pita bread
Quantity: ½ pita
Middle Eastern salad (hold
  olives and feta cheese; request
  lemon wedges or vinegar)
Quantity: 1–2 cups
Kafta (eat half)
Quantity: 3–4 oz
Rice pilaf
Quantity: 1 cup
**Steamed vegetable
  combination**
Quantity: ½ cup
Mineral water
Quantity: unlimited

Estimated	821 calories
Nutrient	36% calories as fat
Evaluation	19% calories as protein
	45% calories as carbohydrate
	88 mg cholesterol
	1010 mg sodium

12

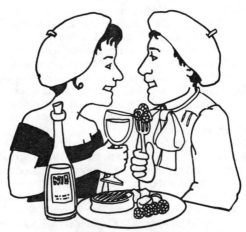

Healthier eating out

French/
Continental
Style

Toaday, the menu selections in continental restaurants offer a wider gamut of choices than ever before. Ingredients and resulting dishes are of multiple ethnic origins, and there's wide variety in the style and healthfulness of food preparation. In most large cities people still find some classic French restaurants continuing to prepare food in the old methods of *haute cuisine*. You'll taste the familiar rich sauces—béchamel, béarnaise, and mornay. But as we enter the 1990s, more and more of the upper-crust restaurants are serving the newer French cuisine, labeled *nouvelle cuisine*.

This is a lighter and healthier French cooking style. You'll see a more in-depth discussion of "French Cuisine: Then and Now" further along in this chapter.

Along with the arrival of nouvelle cuisine, there has been an onslaught of continental dining spots specializing in grilled foods. They offer a variety of grilled, Cajun, and blackened dishes. There are also many upscale restaurants serving the fare of other continental European countries. For instance, fine Italian restaurants serve elegant pasta, veal, and seafood dishes. (See Chapter 7: "Healthier Eating Out: Italian Style.") Though less common, paella is just one Spanish dish that can be ordered in many Spanish dining spots, and Wiener schnitzel is a standard in fine German restaurants.

It's actually quite interesting to reflect on the evolution of continental dining in the United States. To a large extent, several generations ago the foods and preparation methods used by the classic French chefs defined fine dining. For several reasons, that has drastically changed. For some French chefs, there has been an evolution toward the lighter style French cuisine. Due to modern transportation, many more chefs and people alike travel, both nationally and internationally. People are exposed to foods from all over the world. In addition, people from a wider range of countries have emigrated to the U.S. and brought with them their cooking techniques and ingredients. For instance, the uniqueness of Southeast Asian cookery has impacted on dishes served both in American and French restaurants. All of these unique qualities have blended into the "melting pot" of foods available today in America's continental restaurants.

Lastly, there's definitely a wave afoot toward healthier eating. The newer cooking methods—grilling, stir-frying, blackening, poaching—avoid the fat from butter, eggs, and cream, items previously used in large volume in haute cuisine. The newer preparation methods and the use of healthier ingredients illustrate how the great chefs are assisting us in continuing to enjoy great foods while encouraging lower-fat, calorie-conscious dining.

So as the world in a sense becomes smaller due to modern transportation and because America has welcomed people from a broad array of ethnic, cultural, and regional backgrounds, we have ended up with a delightul range of menu listings in gourmet dining spots. Although you can still find strictly French or Italian restaurants, many continental dining spots across the country do not specialize in just one cuisine. These places offer very eclectic menus. For example, there's a very interesting, relatively new restaurant in Boston called Rocco's. Their menu epitomizes eclectic, ranging from seafood fettucini, which sounds quite Italian, to Mexican stuffed shrimp to moo shi duck and chilled beet borscht. This menu takes you around the world!

There are also more upscale restaurants specializing in various American regional cuisines. For instance, California has a style of cuisine that is unique to that area but quickly spreading east. California has also been a leader in introducing diners to new, lighter fare. "California Cuisine" makes use of newer ingredients—sun-dried tomatoes, roasted peppers, cilantro, and interesting herbs—items that blend well with nouvelle cuisine as well as classic French, Mexican, and Italian cooking methods. I recently visited the Piret M Bistro, a restaurant just outside of San Diego. Their menu lists items such as pureed lentil soup, quiche Lorraine, grilled calamari steak, and shrimp with tomato, garlic, and herb sauce. I asked one of the owners if he would define the restaurant as California-French. He said that was an apt description. So again we see a blending of multiple cuisines.

Southwest regional cookery is catching on with its offerings of black bean soup, blue corn polenta, smoked tomatoes, chipotle, and cilantro sauces. Even Italian cuisine has changed over the last ten years. It's lighter, with more pesto sauces and primavera entrees. There's also more Cajun food being served. You now find many restaurants, à la Paul Prudhomme, the well-known New Orleans chef, solely dedicated to serving the healthier Cajun dishes.

So, all in all, continental dining in America is no longer defined by classic French cuisine. There's a wide variety of restaurant choices as well as a wide selection within the menus listings. Also, healthier food preparation (at least in a few dishes) is quickly becoming the order of the day. That makes it easier, though not a snap by any means, for those wishing to eat and stay healthier.

French cuisine then and now

Since French cuisine has played such an important role in defining dining in the world, it's interesting to recap its recent history. Many changes have occurred during the twentieth century. The changes toward the use of healthier ingredients and food preparation methods are more than just a fad. Nouvelle cuisine is here to stay.

One of the qualities that defined classic French cookery, also referred to as *grande* or *haute cuisine,* was its complicated and labor-intensive sauces. The sauces were started with stock and simmered for hours. Many of the sauces contained butter, eggs, cream, and flour to thicken. Béarnaise, béchamel, Bordelaise, and espagnole were just a few of these complex sauces. Expensive ingredients were commonly used in haute cuisine, such as truffles, pâté de foie gras, and crème fraiche. The master chefs of grand French cuisine blossomed during the nineteenth and early twentieth centuries. Haute cuisine was *the* cuisine of the upper class, obviously not the standard fare.

Different regions of France specialized in growing and/or producing particular ingredients or recipes. For instance, in Brittany and Normandy dairy products were a specialty. Alsace-Lorraine brought us pâté de foie gras and quiche Lorraine; and Provence, which is closer to Italy, was known for its sauce Provençal, made with tomatoes, garlic, and olive oil. Dijon, a city in the Burgundy region, is well known for its mustard, which contains a bit of wine. And Bordeaux, beyond being world-renowned for wine production, can also claim Bordelaise sauce.

Around the middle of the twentieth century, there were some changes brewing in how French chefs were preparing foods. Chefs began to abandon the heavy, complex sauces and high-fat ingredients for lighter, more vegetable-based sauces. More chefs were traveling and bringing back cooking styles that they intermingled with the old ones. The result is commonly referred to as nouvelle cuisine. And these lighter preparation techniques have spread, with the chefs, to American restaurants.

In her book *In Madeleine's Kitchen* by Madeleine Kamman, she sums up the definition. French cooking has been "updated for the twentieth century, simplified quite a bit, rejuvenated by foreign and ethnic ingredients, lightened in texture, by both the adoption of Oriental techniques of cooking and modern man's worry about his arteries and the expanse of his waistline, and truly personalized by each cook or chef . . . exercising his/her own creativity at combining ingredients." French cooking is no less an art form, but the bottom line is that what has evolved is great for the health-conscious diner.

The multiple aspects of continental dining

In this chapter we are discussing restaurants where you really go to "dine." No matter what type of food it is—French, Italian, Spanish, or Cajun—you have different expectations in a "continental" restaurant than when you buzz into a fast food spot or grab a quick hamburger or pizza before or after the movies. These are the restaurants in which you expect to be "waited on," where you expect "white glove" service.

Visits to upscale restaurants are often reserved for special occasions—celebrating a birthday, anniversary, or graduation, just to name a few happy events frequently celebrated around elaborate dining. Also, many business meals are eaten in continental-style establishments.

Unlike the quick-order-and-bring-me-a-check restaurants, you can expect to linger over your meal for two to three hours, enjoying the food and the relaxing environment. In this class of restaurant, you will most likely be greeted with some variety of bread and butter. Often these restaurants have their own special breads, which quickly appear at the table soon after you're seated. It might be garlic bread, popovers, herb rolls, or crackers with a cheese spread.

It's more common in these dining situations to order alcoholic beverages, be it a mixed drink before eating and wine with dinner or simply sipping wine throughout the meal. You might be more likely to top off the dinner with a cordial or Irish coffee. For more information on managing alcoholic beverage choices, consult Chapter 19, "Choosing Beverages: Alcoholic and Non-Alcoholic."

Appetizers are more often included as part of the meal. A salad and the main course, served with a starch and vegetable, are often included in the price of the meal. The serving sizes can be quite excessive. Often the piece of fish, chicken, or beef is double the quantity you need, especialy if you're tightly watching the calorie count. Dessert and a hot beverage are usually the conclusion to one of these meals. Remember, you don't have to eat from "soup to nuts." You can pick and choose which courses you want and which are best avoided. It's smart to avoid price-fixed menus because they just encourage overeating.

All of these factors—the length of time spent around food, dangerous foods lying around the table, the quantity served, more elaborate preparation, higher fat foods, alcohol, and tempting desserts—can make continental dining more difficult. Certainly being successful might take more persistence and just plain "white knuckling" it. The good old strategies of preplanning, portion control, and monitoring your fullness come in handy. One special strategy is to focus on the pleasure of the special occasion and the pleasant environment. Really luxuriate in the ambiance; it helps take the importance off the food and what you are and are not eating.

What to consider before ordering

There is no doubt that you can come up with healthy, low-fat and calorie-conscious menu selections when eating continental cuisine. You certainly will need to ask questions and make special requests in order to get your mission accomplished. Remember, don't go to the restaurant starving, drink plenty of non-caloric liquids, practice out-of-sight, out-of-mind techniques, and use the filling low-calorie foods— salads and clear soups.

Fat is, as usual, the biggest concern when trying to keep a lid on the calories and saturated fat. You can start to ingest fat calories right off the bat from the bread and butter or cheese spread on crackers. Try to avoid these by moving them to another part of the table or ask that they be removed, that is, if your dining partners agree.

Appetizers can be loaded with fats. Melted cheese, cheese sauces, mayonnaise, butter, or cream sauce are frequent additions to seafood or vegetable appetizers. Salads can come loaded with dressings and high-fat ingredients—bacon bits, croutons, and egg. The entree might be high in fat to start with, such as prime rib, or it might be low-calorie shrimp made into a high-calorie dish by stuffing it and drenching it with butter before baking. Obviously, some of the decadent desserts often served in better dining spots aren't exactly classified as low fat.

When ordering, it's important to pay attention to the foods as well as the preparation methods. Keep the Red and Green Flag words in mind. The Red Flag Words will often point out high-fat ingredients or preparation methods. The Green Flag Words will steer you in the low fat direction. Certainly portion control can help lower the fat intake. Don't forget, doggie bags are just as acceptable in fine restaurants as they are when eating Chinese food. You might even get your food wrapped up in aluminum foil in the shape of a duck!

For those monitoring sodium consumption, careful ordering, special requests, and portion control can help you keep the milligrams reasonable. Certainly salt and other high-sodium ingredients are used as flavor enhancers. Watch out for preparation methods that clearly connote high sodium, for example, marinated, broiled in teriyaki sauce *or* or lemon soy sauce. Let the waitperson know that you are concerned about the sodium content of your meal. If you are having an entree that is made to order, such as a steak, they probably will be willing not to add any salt in preparation. Also make those special requests: ask for salad dressing on the side or request that a sauce be served on the side so you can control the amount used. Always remember that you are best off with less adulterated food. For instance, order steamed red bliss potatoes rather than rice pilaf or Delmonico potatoes because they won't have as many high-sodium ingredients added.

Managing the menu

The first question most likely asked by the waitperson will be: "May I bring you something to drink?" Have a plan in mind and know if you and your dining partner(s) will be drinking wine with dinner. This might impact your beverage choice. It might be best to avoid a mixed drink and sip instead some wine or a wine spritzer. Always have a non-caloric beverage by your side so you quench your thirst with it rather than the alcoholic beverage. Don't forget, the calorie content of alcoholic beverages adds up quickly.

On to the appetizers. Appetizers are often laden with fat, but if you want one or feel that it is appropriate in the situation, there are reasonably healthy choices. Keep the Red Flag Words in mind and the portions light. Appetizers are perfect for sharing. And by now you can see that items such as grilled marinated shrimp, grilled asparagus with lemon soy sauce (the sauce can be ordered on the side and used to dip), and vegetable mélange with mustard sauce all appear more acceptable than, for example, mussels au gratin, stuffed mushrooms with cream sauce, and pâté de foie gras with toast points.

The rule of thumb with soups is to avoid the creamy variety and look for the words broth, clear soup, and vegetables. Soup can be a good filler, but you often are met with cream of this or that or French onion soup au gratin, and the fat is sky high. Onion soup without the au gratin (cheese), vegetable soup, cold gazpacho, and consommé are good choices. Those monitoring sodium should probably avoid most soups.

Don't pass by the salads. They can often be ordered instead of a high-fat appetizer. Besides, there are salad offerings that fit into any modified meal plan. Look for the healthy greens and low-calorie vegetables. There are newer ingredients being used in salads, such as jicama, endive, radicchio, and fruits. However, there are also plenty of high-fat ingredients put on even before the dressings. You can request that these be omitted or used sparingly: bacon bits, homemade croutons, avocado, nuts, goat or feta cheese, and Parmesan cheese are just a few. Don't forget to always ask for the dressing on the side, and request the light, oil-based varieties.

Now for the main course. The entree, and most frequently the protein portion of the entree, gets the most attention when you're ordering. Will it be duck, lamb, or seafood? Unfortunately, no matter which entree you chose, you will likely be served an excessive portion, especially if you are closely watching calories or have had some bread, salad, appetizers, or alcoholic beverages already. So portion control of the entree is important. Think about sharing, doggie bags, leaving food on your plate, and other strategies that will prevent overeating.

When you are ordering, think about the protein foods with lower fat, saturated fat, and cholesterol: fish, shellfish, and chicken. Look for preparation methods that are on the Green Flag list—grilled, poached, blackened, steamed, stir-fried—these indicate that limited fat is used in preparation. Even though you start with a healthy protein food such as fish or chicken, it can easily become a nutritional disaster. Consider the description of chicken Kiev: breast of chicken filled with herb butter and cheese garlic, served topped with butter sauce. Compare that with the description of chicken saute: diced chicken breast sauteed with sun-dried tomatoes, herbs, and asparagus in olive oil. Certainly neither item is fat free, but the latter is a better choice.

Just because you know that seafood and chicken are lower-fat protein foods doesn't necessarily mean that red meats and duck are off limits. In fact, sometimes the unadulterated preparation of a filet mignon, sliced breast of duck, and veal or lamb chops makes these relatively smart choices.

If you are ordering beef, stick with the small cuts—"petite," "queen," and "eight-ounce," are the usual words used to describe smaller servings. Obviously, these portions are still more than you need but certainly better than the "king," or 12 to 16-ounce portion. A filet mignon, or tenderloin, is leaner than rib eye, sirloin, prime rib, or porterhouse.

Unfortunately, veal is most often breaded and sauteed prior to cooking. But if a broiled veal chop is available, that's a good choice. Lamb can be quite high in fat, but it is most often broiled or grilled, which doesn't add much fat. Don't forget to trim meats well before eating!

Duck is thought of as quite high in fat, and it definitely is with the skin on. However, with the arrival of nouvelle cuisine preparation, one sees a lot more sliced breast of duck served with fruit sauces. It is often quite lean, and most of the fat is gone.

More and more restaurants are offering vegetarian entree listings. Take a look at these. Many times there is a vegetarian stir-fry that might have an Oriental flair. Or there might be a grilled vegetable entree. However, be careful of the vegetarian entrees that are loaded with high-fat cheese, such as vegetarian lasagne.

The starch is usually included with the entree. Again, look for the unadulterated—sans fat—starches. Baked potato, red bliss potato, brown rice, and rice pilaf are frequently offered. Just make sure to ask that no fat be added. If you want sour cream or butter, control the portion yourself. I recently was surprised after ordering the interesting Hawaiian fish, Ahi, with red bliss potatoes. The potatoes appeared nicely opened—with about a tablespoon of sour cream piled on each! I acted surprised, and the waitperson, upon my request, came back with *unadulterated* red bliss potatoes, to which I added a bit of salt and fresh-ground pepper.

Vegetables are also often included with the entree. You might want to ask how these are prepared. If they are topped with a creamy sauce, request that it be held, or if they are sauteed, maybe yours can be steamed. If you are ordering the vegetables à la carte, look for the grilled, sauteed, steamed, or stir-fried varieties. Watch the hollandaise, butter, and creamy sauces.

Somehow dinners in continental restaurants seem to cry out: "Have some dessert." It's likely due to the specialness of the dining, the lingering over the meal, and, needless to say, the often decadent dessert offerings. If you aren't strictly monitoring calories, fat, or blood sugar level, maybe these situations are meant for splurging on a delicious dessert.

Often, we're simply after a taste of something sweet to end the meal. So try to share a dessert with one or several dining partners. Also, in better restaurants, and with lighter cuisine being served, there are fruits listed on the dessert menu. Many times the strawberries or raspberries are topped with crème fraiche, whipped cream, and/or liqueur of some sort. If anything must top your fruit, you're better off with the liqueur—no fat or cholesterol. You might also find that a cup of coffee with a jigger of liqueur added suits your fancy for something a bit sweet. This strategy can help you keep the calories and fat much lower than splitting a piece of ultra-rich double fudge chocolate cake.

When the menu arrives, look for certain key words and phrases that signal the nutritional advisability of the items. We call them "Green Flag" (go for it) and "Red Flag" (steer clear) words.

Green Flag Words

balsamic vinegar or vinaigrette
cilantro
roasted red peppers
sun-dried tomatoes
blackened
Cajun spiced
wine sauce, red or white (make sure no cream is added)
sauce of tomato, garlic, and spices
wine and herbs
green spices—rosemary, tarragon, basil, oregano

chutney sauce

fruit sauces—mango, raspberry,
orange, apple

roasted

steamed

poached

grilled

marinated

broiled

en brochette

mustard sauce (make sure it's not
a mustard cream sauce)

salsa

available as appetizer portion

half portions available

petite or queen size

**Red Flag
Words**

creamy mushroom sauce

cheese sauce

blended with melted cheese

au gratin

served with drawn butter

stuffed with seasoned
breadcrumbs

stuffed and baked with butter
sauce

butter

cream sauce

garlic and herbed cream sauce

casserole (usually indicates added
fat)

bacon

sausage

blue cheese

wrapped in phyllo dough

wrapped in pastry shell

pistachio, orange, herb, or shallot
butter

hollandaise

mayonnaise-based sauce

sour cream

crème fraiche

Special Requests Continental Style

Could you serve the sauce on the side?

Would you serve the salad dressing on the side?

Could I get some vinegar or lemon wedges for my salad rather than the dressing?

May I have some Dijon mustard for my potato?

Please don't add butter or sour cream to my potato, but bring it on the side.

Please don't bring out the drawn butter, but I will have a good supply of lemon wedges.

Could I ask you how this is prepared?

Is it possible to have these vegetables steamed rather than sauteed?

Please bring my appetizer when you bring the others their main course.

Could we get an extra plate to split this appetizer (or entree)?

Can you bring several extra forks; we are going to split this dessert?

May I have this wrapped up to take home?

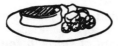

Typical Menu: Continental Style

Appetizers **Mussels au gratin** (mussels in garlic butter sauce with cheese topping)

✓**Shrimp,** marinated and grilled (quarter pound of shrimp marinated in lemon, garlic, and spices and grilled over mesquite chips)

Stuffed mushrooms (prepared with herbs and seasoned breadcrumbs, topped with a blend of rosemary in cream sauce)

Pate de la maison (pâté de foie gras, served with toast points)

Goat cheese (wrapped in Bibb lettuce with sun-dried tomatoes and grilled over mesquite chips)

Escargots (snails served in traditional style, with garlic, herb, butter sauce)

✓**Vegetable melange** with mustard sauce (freshly cut raw vegetables served in a lettuce cup with curry mustard sauce)

✓**Grilled asparagus** with lemon soy sauce (fresh asparagus, grilled and basted in a light oriental sauce)

Artichoke hearts with feta cheese (artichoke hearts marinated and sauteed in olive oil, topped with crumbled feta cheese)

Soups **Soup du jour** (server will describe today's special)

French onion soup (traditional style, rich onion soup, served in a crock with melted cheese)

✓*Preferred Choice*

✓**Jellied consomme** (clear light broth, served chilled)

Cream of spinach soup (creamy soup with fresh steamed spinach)

✓**Gazpacho** (cold tomato-based soup of assorted pureed fresh vegetables)

Salads   ✓**House salad** (mixture of romaine and Bibb lettuce, with red onions, red peppers, and sprouts, served with raspberry vinaigrette dressing)

✓**Marinated tomatoes** (sliced tomatoes marinated with red onions in olive oil and balsamic vinegar, topped with crumbled feta cheese)

✓**Melon salad** with avocado dressing (slices of cantaloupe and honeydew melon, topped with creamy avocado dressing)

✓**Exotic greens** (mixture of radicchio, endive, watercress, and jicama, served with balsamic vinaigrette)

✓**Spinach salad** (fresh spinach, topped with sliced mushrooms, egg, and bacon bits, served with hot bacon dressing)

Entrees   **MEATS***

Beef Wellington (fillet of beef covered with thin layer of goose liver paté and wrapped in flaky pastry shell, topped with Bordelaise sauce)

✓**Petite filet mignon** with mushroom sauce (small fillet broiled to your liking, topped with light sauteed mushroom sauce)

New York sirloin strip steak, 12 ozs (center cut sirloin, broiled to your liking)

Rib eye steak, 12 ozs (aged rib eye, broiled or blackened to your liking)

✓**Marinated pork chop,** 10 ozs (center cut pork chop, marinated and broiled in sherry and lemon herb sauce)

✓**Rack of lamb** (individual rack of lamb, broiled with a glaze of honey mustard sauce)

Veal Oscar (veal cutlet sauteed with lobster meat and asparagus, topped with hollandaise sauce)

POULTRY*

Chicken Kiev (boneless breast of chicken, filled with herb butter and cheese garlic, topped with butter sauce)

✓**Chicken saute** (sliced chicken breast, sauteed with sun-dried tomatoes, asparagus, and herbs in olive oil)

Duck à l'orange (one-half Long Island duckling grilled and basted with orange glaze)

✓**Duck with raspberry sauce** (sliced breast of duck served with light raspberry lemon sauce)

SEAFOOD*

Stuffed shrimp (four jumbo shrimp, stuffed with blend of crab-meat and seasoned breadcrumbs, baked and basted with garlic butter sauce)

✓**Poached salmon** with smoked tomato sauce and cilantro (salmon fillet, lightly poached in wine and topped with delicate tomato and cilantro sauce)

Dover sole in champagne cream sauce (dover sole, baked in a light champagne-based cream sauce)

✓**Blackened tuna** served with mango chutney sauce

*All above entrees served with choice of rice pilaf, baked potato, steamed red bliss potatoes, or fried potato puffs.

PASTA

Seafood fettucini (shrimp and scallops, topped with basil cream sauce)

Cheese-stuffed tortellini topped with sauteed broccoli and mushrooms

VEGETARIAN

✓**Oriental stir-fry** (fresh garden vegetables, stir-fried in olive oil, Tamari, garlic, and lemon, served over brown rice)

Vegetables ✓**Squash and zucchini,** sauteed in lemon herb butter

✓**Snow peas,** sauteed with red pepper

Creamed spinach

✓**Asparagus,** steamed and topped with hollandaise sauce

Desserts ✓**Strawberries** topped with crème fraiche

Key lime pie (lightly sweetened graham cracker crust filled with tart Key lime mousse)

Peanut butter cheesecake (New York-style rich cheesecake with a hint of peanut butter flavor)

Chocolate raspberry cake (double fudge cake, iced and filled with raspberry jam)

✓**Fresh raspberries** topped with Chambord liqueur

Now that you've seen what may be available on the menu, look over the following five "Model Meals" for suggestions on how to order to achieve specific nutritional goals. Models are numbered one to five for quick reference, and each is followed by an "Estimated Nutrient Evaluation" that analyzes the content of that meal.

May I Take Your Order

Healthy	30% Calories as fat
Daily	20% Calories as protein
Eating	50% Calories as carbohydrate
Goals	300 mg/day Cholesterol
	3000 mg/day Sodium

Low Calorie/ Low Fat Model Meal

Shrimp, marinated and grilled (listed as appetizer but request as main course)
Quantity: 1 order
Exchanges: 3 meat (lean); 1 fat

Exotic greens (dressing on the side)
Quantity: 1–2 cups
Exchanges: 1–2 vegetable

Balsamic vinaigrette dressing (on the side)
Quantity: 1 tbsp
Exchanges: 1 fat

Red bliss potatoes, steamed (request no butter)
Quantity: 2
Exchanges: 2 starch

Strawberries (hold crème fraiche)
Quantity: ½ cup
Exchanges: 1 fruit

Wine
Quantity: 6 oz
Exchanges: account for calories but don't omit exchanges

Estimated	581 calories
Nutrient	20% calories as fat
Evaluation	23% calories as protein
	40% calories as carbohydrate

17% calories as alcohol
166 mg cholesterol
650 mg sodium

**❷
Low Calorie/
Low
Cholesterol
Model Meal**

Gazpacho
Quantity: 1 cup
Blackened tuna (chutney sauce
  on the side)
Quantity: 4 oz (½ order)
Baked potato
Quantity: 1
Sour cream for above
Quantity: 2 tbsp
Snow peas with red peppers
Quantity: 1 cup
Mineral water
Quantity: unlimited

Estimated
Nutrient
Evaluation

589 calories
32% calories as fat
27% calories as protein
41% calories as carbohydrate
  72 mg cholesterol
670 mg sodium

**❸
Higher
Calorie/Low
Fat Model
Meal**

House salad (dressing on the
  side)
Quantity: 1–2 cups
Exchanges: 1–2 vegetables
Raspberry vinaigrette dressing
  (on the side)
Quantity: 2 tbsp
Exchanges: 2 fat
Petite filet mignon
Quantity: 3 oz (½ order)
Exchanges: 3 meat (med.)

Red bliss potatoes, steamed (request no butter)
Quantity: 1 medium
Exchanges: 1 starch
Oriental stir-fry with brown rice
Quantity: ½ order
Exchanges: 2 fat; 2 vegetable; 2 starch
Fresh raspberries with Chambord
Quantity: ½ cup
Exchanges: 1 fruit; account for calories but don't omit exchanges for alcohol

Estimated Nutrient Evaluation	858 calories
	32% calories as fat
	18% calories as protein
	44% calories as carbohydrate
	6% calories as alcohol
	67 mg cholesterol
	790 mg sodium

❹
Higher Calorie/Low Cholesterol Model Meal

Marinated tomatoes
Quantity: 1 order
Chicken saute
Quantity: 1 order
Rice pilaf
Quantity: 1 cup
Key lime pie
Quantity: ½ piece

Estimated Nutrient Evaluation	888 calories
	36% calories as fat
	23% calories as protein
	41% calories as carbohydrate
	188 mg cholesterol
	1350 mg sodium

Low Sodium Model Meal

Spinach salad (hold dressing)
Quantity: 1–2 cups
Balsamic vinegar (special request; on the side)
Quantity: unlimited
Duck with raspberry sauce
Quantity: 4 oz (½ order)
Baked potato
Quantity: 1 large
Butter for above
Quantity: 1 pat
Asparagus (hold hollandaise sauce and order lemon wedges)
Quantity: 1 cup
Coffee
Quantity: unlimited
Amaretto liqueur
Quantity: 1½ oz

Estimated Nutrient Evaluation

827 calories
28% calories as fat
22% calories as protein
41% calories as carbohydrate
9% calories as alcohol
124 mg cholesterol
550 mg sodium

13

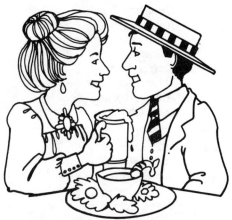

Healthier eating out

American Style

A t mid-priced restaurants serving so-called
"American fare" the order may be a mushroom cheeseburger with French fries, chef
salad served in a fried tortilla shell, or a
teriyaki-style chicken breast served with
rice and sauteed vegetables. These restaurants are
best defined as a few steps up from the fast food stops
and a few steps down from continental cuisine, featuring cloth napkins, flowers, music, and—particularly—
ambiance.

American style eating spots are frequented by people wishing to sit and relax, be served quickly, and

simply unwind from a busy day. These restaurants fit the bill for lunch or dinner. They're great places to meet friends or family, for lunch or after work, to drop by before or after the movies, to get a late night snack, or to use if you just don't feel like cooking.

American style restaurants line America's highways and city streets, and a number of them belong to major restaurant chains. Often these businesses have locations across the country, or they concentrate on one or two regions. Some of the popular ones are T.G.I. Friday's, Bennigan's, and Houlihan's. Others, well known across the country, include Denny's, Howard Johnson's, and the Ground Round, just to name a few.

Independently owned restaurants located around the country also serve "American fare." Their menus have many similar offerings to the popular chains. Common entries are nachos, buffalo chicken wings, burgers with toppings, and pasta, chef, or Greek salads. Generally, no matter what city or town you're in, an American style restaurant is just around the corner.

What's offered in American style restaurants?

Though we call these "American style" restaurants, what is American fare? The menus generally reflect a melting pot of multiple cuisines. American fare is ultimately a blending of foods from different cultures with American adaptations. On the menus you'll find echoes of multiple ethnic cuisines, especially the most popular – Mexican, Italian, and Oriental. For instance, the menu from T.G.I. Friday's includes fajitas from Mexico, almond chicken from the Orient, baked manicotti from Italy, and blackened Cajun chicken from the Bayou country. As other ethnic cuisines become more popular, we'll probably start to see those items appear on the menus of "American" restaurants, too. Look for the Thai appetizer satay and Indian offerings of curried chicken and shrimp in the near future.

Obviously, some of the selections on these menus are hardly ideal when viewed in terms of healthy eating goals. Fried mozzarella sticks, quiche Lorraine, fried shrimp tempura, or a Philadelphia cheese steak are just a sampling of the usual high-fat and calories offerings.

Burgers, available with a variety of toppings, ranging from cheese to bacon or sauteed vegetables, are
available at most American restaurants. Consider the
calorie count in a four-ounce cooked hamburger (and
that's a comparatively small one) served on a roll with
French fries and a house salad with Thousand Island
dressing. This meal adds up to slightly over 800
calories, with almost 45 percent of the calories coming from fat. That's a bit off the mark of our 30 percent fat goal.

But by no means should these restaurants be
avoided. There are good choices, and where there's a
will, there's a way. For instance, peel-and-eat shrimp
are often available as an appetizer. Blackened or Cajun chicken, either on a salad, as a dinner, or served
on a sandwich roll, seem to be appearing more frequently on these menus. Often, you'll see stir-fry
dishes or a broiled fish dinner. These are just a scat-
tering of many healthy choices often available. As eating healthier becomes a more important goal for all
Americans, more menu offerings will, hopefully, reflect the desire to keep fat, cholesterol, calories, and
sodium controlled.

However, we've got a long way to go before these
menus list many healthy selections. It will be great
to see several healthier appetizers, half or smaller portions available at lower prices, and more low-fat or
no-oil salad dressings. But for the next few years at
least, you'll have to maneuver your way through the
mine field of high-fat and high-calorie menu listings
when eating American fare.

What to consider before ordering

As usual, the same watchwords for healthy dining
apply. Plan ahead, make smart menu choices, and
watch those portions. Think about what you will order prior to arriving at the restaurant. Chances are
you have eaten at this restaurant before. You have
a good sense of what's on the menu and which are your
best bets. If possible, don't tempt your taste buds by
looking at the mouth-watering choices on the often
extensive bill of fare.

If you choose to peruse the menu, remember that
fat is the number one enemy in these restaurants. Be
wary of the preparation methods as well as the fats
that are added. When monitoring the fat content of

your selection, watch for the Red Flag Words that ring out "FAT, FAT, FAT," such as "fried," "breaded and fried," and "topped with melted cheese." Look for the Green Flag Words that ring out "LEAN, LEAN, LEAN," such as "broiled," "blackened," and "with vegetables." Watch for extra fats, for example, mayonnaise spread on sandwich bread or butter smeared on a hamburger bun before heating or grilling. Try to stick with the low-fat sandwich spreads such as mustard, horseradish, and Mexican hot sauce. Make the waitperson aware that you are concerned about extra fats. Be specific and assertive about special requests.

Don't forget that the mixed salads—tuna, chicken, seafood, or egg—are often chock full of mayonnaise. The unadulterated items are better—turkey, chicken, or roast beef. If you're ordering a sandwich, avoid croissants—they're loaded with fat. Go with a roll, whole-wheat bread, or a pita pocket. Also be aware of what is served with the meal. For instance, if the accompaniment is French fries, try to order a baked potato, a side of rice pilaf, or sauteed vegetables instead.

The next challenge is to avoid overeating. To accomplish this goal, practice several ordering strategies. Unfortunately, the portions are usually larger than necessary. Some restaurants will offer soup or salad with a half-sandwich. That portion may be just enough, especially if calories are your chief concern. Also, if you are dining with someone, consider splitting two entrees. For example, one person orders a hamburger and fries and the other orders a Greek salad or an appetizer of vegetables and dip. Another strategy is not to order an entree but piece together appetizers, such as peel-and-eat shrimp, a bowl of chili, and a baked potato and/or salad and roll to make a complete meal. Don't feel compelled to order an entree. These tactics reduce the amount of food in front of you. This is a first step, and possibly the most important, toward not overeating.

Managing the menu

Appetizers present a big problem. On American style restaurant menus the crunchy, munchy, fried appetizers are often hard to resist, but they are deadly in terms of fat and calorie content. Frequent offerings

are nachos or super nachos, fried tortilla chips with
more high-fat items loaded on top—cheese, sour
cream, and guacamole. Other appetizers that add insult to injury are fried mozzarella sticks, buffalo
chicken wings, which are traditionally dipped in blue
cheese dressing, and potato skins, which are first fried
and then loaded with cheese, bacon bits, and sour
cream.

A few redeeming choices are shrimp cocktail, peel-
and-eat shrimp served with cocktail sauce, and, at the
occasional raw bar, combinations of oysters, shrimp,
and clams. A vegetable dip platter might be listed.
Unfortunately, the dip will be 100 percent fat, but
there is an alternative. Ask for a side of the low-calorie
salad dressing and use that for a low-fat dip.

If your dining partners are ordering high-fat appetizers, try ordering a house salad or healthy soup
as your appetizer. That's easier than trying to avoid
eating the tasty little fried items once they greet you
at the table.

Soup listings in American style restaurants don't
commonly offer many choices to the health-conscious
diner. It's usual to find French onion topped with
cheese, New England clam chowder, and several
creamy or cheesy soups. Often there is a soup of the
day, which might be a broth-based Manhattan clam
chowder or a gumbo. These are fine choices unless sodium is a concern. Prepared soups are all too frequently loaded with salt.

When considering an entree, you'll encounter many
mouth-watering choices. You'll find a number of salad
offerings, sandwiches, burgers with various toppings,
and hot entrees accompanied with rice, potato, and/or
some vegetable combination. Healthy selections are
available in each of these categories. If you can't decide exactly what you want before looking at the
menu, maybe you can at least narrow it down to the
food category. That way you can limit menu
"shopping."

The salad choices on American fare menus have
really expanded over the last few years. This is great
for the health-conscious diner, but you still must be
careful to observe what is topped onto that bed of
mixed greens. It's common to find a house salad, Cobb
salad, taco salad, chicken or tuna salad on a bed of
vegetables, chef, Greek, and spinach salads. Some
restaurants serve many of their dinner salads in fried

tortilla shells. You are best off asking that yours be served without the shell. They are just too tempting to have sitting in front of you.

When choosing a salad, observe the Red and Green Flag Words. Often many items are included, some great and some not. Let's consider the Cobb salad: on top of a mixture of greens you find chicken breast, crsip bacon, avocado, Cheddar cheese, hard-boiled egg, black olives, tomatoes, and sprouts. This is quite a mixture of Red and Green Flag ingredients. If it's Cobb salad you want, simply request that a few items be omitted. For instance, "please hold the crisp bacon, Cheddar cheese, and hard-boiled egg and replace them with a few more tomatoes and sprouts."

So read the ingredients carefully, and request what you want in and out of your salad. An important consideration is the dressing. First and foremost, it should always be ordered on the side. Many times these restaurants stock a light dressing or oil and vinegar. Don't forget about lemon wedges. Also, if there are Mexican menu listings, there will be Mexican hot sauce to use as a zesty salad dressing. Refer to Chapter 15, "Healthier Eating Out: Salad Bar Style," for more details about and suggestions for salad dressings.

Sandwiches are commonly listed on American fare menus—some healthy and some not. Unfortunately, they are frequently served with an excessive portion of protein. Half a sandwich with soup, salad, or a baked potato will be plenty for most of us. Another problem with sandwiches is that they are frequently served with French fries or potato chips and a bit of creamy coleslaw. These accompaniments are loaded with fat and can significantly raise the calories. You are best advised not to have these presented to you on the plate. Either request that they be left off and replaced by a healthier offering, or see if a fellow dining partner would be interested in taking them off your hands.

When focusing on the sandwiches, it's again important to observe the multiple ingredients. Are they healthy or loaded with fat? Some of the healthier sandwiches are among the charbroiled, blackened, and teriyaki chicken breast listings. A French dip, roast beef, ham, or turkey sandwich is acceptable. If you've got a few more calories to spare, the tuna or seafood salad is OK.

American Style

Sandwich offerings to avoid are the Reuben, Philadelphia cheese steak, clubs, and melts. Unfortunately, many sandwiches start off sounding healthy, but high-fat ingredients are piled on top. So all you have to do is make those special requests. The cheese, mayonnaise, special (high-fat) sauces, crisp bacon, and/or avocado can always be left off. Don't forget about using the low-calorie sandwich spreads and other sauces that you see elsewhere on the menu—mustard, low calorie salad dressings, Mexican hot sauce, barbecue sauce, horseradish (great on a French dip), and honey mustard sauce (great with chicken) are just a few.

On to one of American's favorite foods—burgers. Hamburgers with various toppings seem to be a constant on these menus. The quantity of meat is usually larger than necessary, but in some places you have a choice of a regular or jumbo patty. Always choose the smaller portion. Even that size will be more protein and fat than you need. If the quantity of meat is noted, for instance, "six ounces or a half-pound of first quality ground meat," remember that it is based on the raw quantity used. So it does cook down by one or two ounces. A six-ounce hamburger will result in a cooked serving of between four and five ounces.

Often the hamburger toppings are among the Red Flag Words—melted cheese, bacon, blue cheese, or guacamole. However, there are also reasonable choices such as sauteed onions, green peppers and/or mushrooms, sliced lettuce, tomato, onions, jalapeño peppers, and barbecue sauce. Pick and choose the healthy toppings.

Sometimes hot entrees are avoided because we think of the salads or sandwiches as lighter or lower-calorie meals. Interestingly, several of the hot entree items turn out to be healthier choices. Again, there are some nutritional disasters lurking. You'll find many fried items and those topped with Red Flag ingredients. If you skirt around these, you're likely to find a stir-fry dish or two, a broiled fresh fish, fajitas, teriyaki, or blackened chicken, fish, or beef.

Many times you'll have to open your mouth and make *several* special requests about adding or deleting items. American style restaurants love to pile on high-fat ingredients. Also be careful to check the accompaniments. French fries are commonly served but may easily be replaced by a baked potato, sauteed vegetables, or rice pilaf.

In the way of beverages, make sure you always have a glass of water in front of you. Drink plenty of fluids—it's good for you and also helps fill you up and not out. Many American style restaurants serve alcohol. If your meal plan allows, you might want to consider enjoying an alcoholic beverage. These restaurants often list milk under beverages, but find out if it's low fat or skim. Additional beverages should come from the non-caloric choices: mineral water, club soda, diet tonic water, or sugar-free carbonated beverages. For further details on beverages, consult Chapter 19, "Choosing Beverages: Alcoholic and Non-Alcoholic."

Desserts in these restaurants are best passed by. The most frequent offerings seem to be cheesecake, some deadly rich chocolate cake, apple pie, ice cream pies, sundaes, or simply several scoops of ice cream. Once in a while you'll see fruit sorbet listed, which is a decent choice but by no means low cal.

The best of the worst dessert choices would be fruit pie, without the à la mode or whipped cream, ice cream, or sorbet ordered with at least a couple of spoons. Though I haven't seen it yet, my prediction is that someday soon we'll see frozen yogurt, now becoming increasingly popular, served in American style restaurants. Non-fat frozen yogurt will be a better dessert choice for those with diabetes, people monitoring saturated fat in order to lower their blood cholesterol, and those watching total calories—that includes just about everyone!

When the menu arrives, look for certain key words and phrases that signal the nutritional advisability of the items. We call them "Green Flag" (go for it) and "Red Flag" (steer clear) words.

Green Flag Words

sauteed onions, peppers, and/or mushrooms
jalapeños
BBQ sauce (watch sugar content)
cocktail sauce
teriyaki sauce
honey mustard (watch sugar content)
mustard (Dijon, Pommery)
crisp lettuce and/or sliced tomatoes

green or red onion
spicy Mexican beef or chicken
blackened
mesquite-grilled
with oriental sauce
charbroiled
marinated and broiled
stir-fry
Cajun sauce
barbecued
low-calorie salad dressing

Red Flag Words

cheese (grated, melted, topped with, smothered in)
guacamole
bacon (strips, crisp, crumbled)
golden fried
crispy fried
deep-fried
lightly fried
battered and fried
sour cream
loaded with cheese, bacon, and/or sour cream
blue cheese (crumbled, topped with, or salad dressing)
rolled in breadcrumbs and fried
butter
creamy garlic butter
served in crisp tortilla shell
served on crispy nachos
sausage
large, jumbo, piled high, stacked
Alfredo sauce
cream sauce
mayonnaise, garlic mayonnaise, mayonnaise-based sauce

**Special
Requests
American
Style**

Please bring my House Salad when you bring the others their appetizers.

I'd like to order an appetizer as my main course. But will you bring it when you bring the others their entrees?

Please put the salad dressing on the side.

On the blackened chicken sandwich, please leave off the cheese.

On the roast beef sandwich, can you make sure they don't put any butter or mayonnaise on the bread? However, I'd like a side of mustard or horseradish.

Please bring some vinegar or lemon wedges for me to use on my salad.

Do you have Mexican hot sauce? Could I get a bit to use on my salad?

Please hold the sour cream, but you can load on the lettuce and tomato.

Please bring me a little bowl of low-calorie dressing that I can use for the vegetable dip.

Could I substitute a baked potato for the French fries?

I know the sandwich or hamburger comes with French fries, but could you leave them off the plate?

Could I get that sandwich served on whole-wheat bread rather than on a croissant?

We are going to split the salad and the hamburger, so could you bring an extra plate?

May I have the rest of this wrapped up to take home?

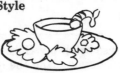

Typical Menu: American Style

Appetizers **Nachos** (nacho chips covered with melted Monterey Jack cheese and jalapeño peppers, served with Mexican hot sauce)

Super nachos (nacho chips covered with melted Monterey Jack cheese, refried beans, spicy beef or chicken, shredded lettuce, and tomatoes, served with Mexican hot sauce)

Buffalo chicken wings (marinated chicken wings in hot and spicy sauce, lightly fried, and served with blue cheese dressing and celery sticks)

✓**Peel-and-eat shrimp** (one-quarter pound boiled shrimp in a spicy sauce, served with cocktail sauce)

Potato skins (fried and crispy potato skins, filled with cheese and your choice of bacon bits, sour cream, and/or onions)

Mozzarella sticks (sticks of mozzarella cheese, rolled in breadcrumbs and fried; served with marinara sauce)

✓**Raw bar platter** (combination of oysters on the halfshell, steamed littleneck clams, and jumbo shrimp, served with cocktail sauce)

Chicken fingers (small pieces of tender chicken breast breaded and fried, served with choice of honey mustard or barbecue sauce)

✓*Preferred Choice*

Soups

New England clam chowder
(creamy New England style chowder with chunks of clams and potato, served with oyster crackers)

French onion soup (crock of rich onion soup, smothered with Swiss cheese)

✓**Chili** (spicy mixture of pinto beans, ground beef, and sauteed onions and peppers, topped with onions and Monterey Jack cheese)

✓**Vegetable gumbo** (blend of garden vegetables, onions, tomatoes, broccoli, and green beans simmered in Cajun spices)

Salads

✓**House salad** (blend of greens, with sliced cucumbers and tomatoes, topped with alfalfa sprouts; choice of dressings)

✓**Spinach salad** (fresh spinach topped with sliced mushrooms, eggs, bacon bits, and croutons, served with hot bacon dressing)

✓**Seafood pasta salad** (rotini blended with baby shrimp and red pepper, tossed with Italian dressing, and served on bed of mixed greens)

✓**Blackened chicken salad** (slices of marinated and blackened chicken breast, served with mixed salad greens, avocado slices, cherry tomatoes, and broccoli florets, topped with shredded Swiss cheese and croutons)

✓**Mexican salad** (choice of spicy chicken or beef, served on bed of mixed greens, with spicy Mexican beans, red and green peppers, tomato, and Monterey Jack cheese, all in crispy flour tortilla shell)

✓**Chef salad** (julienne sliced turkey, ham, and Swiss cheese, served on bed of lettuce greens, diced tomatoes, red and green pepper rounds, all in crispy flour tortilla shell)

Choice of Salad Dressings:

House (creamy garlic)	Thousand Island
	Hot bacon
	✓Lemon vinaigrette
✓Italian	✓Oil and vinegar
French	✓Low-calorie Italian
Blue cheese	Ranch

**Sand-
wiches***

Philadelphia cheese steak (thinly sliced beef, grilled with onions and mushrooms, and topped with melted cheese; served in submarine roll)

✓**French dip** (thinly sliced beef, topped with melted provolone cheese, and served in submarine roll with natural gravy)

✓**Blackened chicken sandwich** (breast of chicken marinated and blackened on the grill, topped with lettuce, tomato, sprouts, crisp bacon slices, and Cheddar cheese)

Tuna melt (creamy tuna salad, topped with melted Swiss cheese and served with lettuce and tomato)

Seafood salad croissant (flaky croissant filled with mixture of creamy seafood salad, celery, and onions, served with lettuce and tomato)

*All sandwiches are served with French fries and creamy coleslaw

Burgers*

Regular hamburgers are 6 ozs. of ground beef and jumbo size are 9 ozs.

✓**American hamburger**
Cheeseburger (add slice of Swiss or Cheddar cheese)
Bacon cheeseburger (add several slices of bacon and slice of Monterey Jack cheese)
✓**Veggie burger** (add sauteed onions, peppers, and mushrooms)
Chili burger (add spicy Mexican chili)

*All burgers are served with sliced tomato on bed of lettuce, with French fries and side dish of creamy coleslaw

Hot Entrees

✓**Fajitas** (choice of chicken or beef, grilled with sliced onions and green peppers, served with warm flour tortillas and sides of sour cream, guacamole, Mexican hot sauce)
Baby back ribs (robust portion of pork ribs, marinated and barbecued with zesty barbecue sauce, and served with fried onion rings and baked beans)
✓**Teriyaki chicken breast** (boneless breast marinated in teriyaki sauce and grilled; served with rice pilaf and sauteed vegetables)
Chicken fried steak (sirloin steak, dipped in batter, and fried; served with country gravy, baked potato, and steamed vegetables)
✓**Oriental stir-fry** (choice of chicken, shrimp, or just vegetables, stir-fried with oriental sauces, and served over a bed of Chinese egg noodles)

           Fettuccini primavera (sauteed broccoli, mushrooms, and red peppers, tossed with creamy Alfredo sauce, and served on bed of fettucini)

Combina-   ✓**Soup and salad** (bowl of any
tions   soup and house salad)
           Quiche and salad (slice of ham, broccoli, and mushroom quiche, served with house salad)
           ✓**Soup and half sandwich** (bowl of any soup, served with half of French dip or seafood salad sandwich)
           ✓**Salad and half sandwich** (house salad, served with half of French dip or seafood salad sandwich)

Side   **French fries**
Orders   **Creamy coleslaw**
           ✓**Rice pilaf**
           ✓**Baked potato** with choice of butter and/or sour cream
           ✓**Sauteed vegetables**

Desserts   **Mud pie** (chocolate graham cracker crust filled with coffee ice cream and topped with fudge sauce)
           ✓**Deep-dish apple pie** à la mode (vanilla ice cream) or topped with whipped cream
           New York style cheesecake (topped with choice of strawberry or blueberry sauce)
           Ice cream (two scoops of vanilla, chocolate, or strawberry)
           Hot fudge sundae (two scoops of vanilla ice cream, topped with hot fudge sauce, walnuts, and whipped cream)
           ✓**Sorbet** (two scoops of raspberry or lemon sherbet)

Now that you've seen what may be available on the menu, look over the following five "Model Meals" for suggestions on how to order to achieve specific nutritional goals. Models are numbered one to five for quick reference, and each is followed by an "Estimated Nutrient Evaluation" that analyzes the content of that meal.

May I Take Your Order

Healthy	30% Calories as fat
Daily	20% Calories as protein
Eating	50% Calories as carbohydrate
Goals	300 mg/day Cholesterol
	3000 mg/day Sodium

❶

Low Calorie/   **Peel-and-eat shrimp**
Low Fat   *Quantity:* 1 order (9-12 med.)
Model Meal   *Exchanges:* 3 meat (lean)
              Cocktail sauce for above
              Quantity: 2 tbsp
              Exchanges: free
              Oriental stir-fry, vegetable
              Quantity: 1½ cups
              Exchanges: 2 fat; 3 vegetable
              Chinese egg noodles with above
              Quantity: 1 cup
              Exchanges: 2 starch
              Sorbet, raspberry (split order)
              Quantity: ¾ cup
              Exchanges: ½ fat; 1 starch; 1 fruit
              Mineral water
              Quantity: unlimited
              Exchanges: free

Estimated	608 calories
Nutrient	21% calories as fat
Evaluation	21% calories as protein
	58% calories as carbohydrate
	227 mg cholesterol (high, due to shrimp)
	970 mg sodium

❷
Low Calorie/ **Chili** (hold the cheese)
Low *Quantity:* 1 cup
Cholesterol **House salad** (dressing on the side)
Model Meal *Quantity:* 2 cups
Italian dressing (low calorie)
Quantity: 2 tbsp
Baked potato (hold butter and
sour cream; use chili to dress)
Quantity: 1 large
Light beer
Quantity: 12 oz

Estimated   595 calories
Nutrient   17% calories as fat
Evaluation 24% calories as protein
46% calories as carbohydrate
13% calories as alcohol
135 mg cholesterol
1146 mg sodium

❸
Higher **House salad** (dressing on the side)
Calorie/Low *Quantity:* 2 cups
Fat Model *Exchanges:* 2 vegetable
Meal **Blue cheese dressing** (request
vinegar)
Quantity: 1 tbsp
Exchanges: 1 fat
Teriyaki chicken breast
Quantity: 4 oz
Exchanges: 4 meat (lean)
Rice pilaf
Quantity: 1 cup
Exchanges: 3 starch
Sauteed vegetables
Quantity: 1 cup
Exchanges: 1 fat; 2 vegetable
Wine
Quantity: 1 glass (6 oz)
Exchanges: account for calories
but don't omit exchanges

Estimated Nutrient Evaluation	758 calories 31% calories as fat 22% calories as protein 32% calories as carbohydrate 15% calories as alcohol 120 mg cholesterol 1170 mg sodium

❹

Higher Calorie/Low Cholesterol Model Meal	**Blackened chicken salad** (hold cheese; request more tomatoes and broccoli; request Mexican hot sauce) *Quantity:* 1 order **Lemon vinaigrette dressing** *Quantity:* 2 tbsp **Dinner roll** *Quantity:* 1 **Deep-dish apple pie a la mode** (hold ice cream; ask for 2 forks and extra plate) *Quantity:* ½ piece

Estimated Nutrient Evaluation	795 calories 35% calories as fat 19% calories as protein 46% calories as carbohydrate 157 mg cholesterol 1080 mg sodium

❺

Low Sodium Model Meal	**Veggie burger** (hold French fries and coleslaw) *Quantity:* 1 (4½ oz cooked) **Baked potato** (hold butter and sour cream; request mustard) *Quantity:* 1 large

Dijon mustard for above
Quantity: 1–2 tbsp
Milk (low fat or skim)
Quantity: 8 oz

Estimated   805 calories
Nutrient   34% calories as fat
Evaluation   27% calories as protein
              39% calories as carbohydrate
              130 mg cholesterol
              874 mg sodium

14

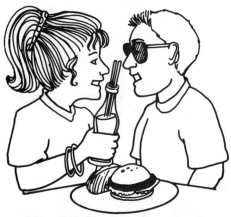

Healthier eating out

Fast Food Style

Many people believe the idea of eating a healthy meal at any fast food restaurant is simply an impossibility. The thought of fast foods brings images of cheeseburgers, French fries, shakes, and fried fruit pies—hardly items that fall into the healthy and nutritious category. But even though we've supposedly become more nutrition conscious, people continue to flock to fast food stops. The dollars spent on fast food continue to escalate, and the number of outlets around the country, for that matter around the world, multiply exponentially.

The fast food business has certainly benefited from our 1980's "the quicker the better" mentality. We want to do everything fast, including eating. The fast food business began in earnest in the 1940s–1950s. Growth became more rapid through the 1970s and 1980s, as society continued to demand a more rapid pace. As long as the ideal of getting things done quickly continues to be of paramount importance, fast food will have a place in the American diet.

Over the last several years, as Americans have become more health conscious, fast food outlets have taken a dose of criticism. They have been criticized about the quality of their products, the high fat nature of the foods, and the types of fats used. In some ways they have responded well to the harsh criticism. Over the last five to ten years, it has become possible to purchase salads, low-fat or skim milk, or a baked potato. Healthwise, this certainly beats the limited choices of hamburgers, fried chicken, French fries, and shakes.

Interestingly, some of the internationally recognized chains have responded to consumers' health demands more quickly than many expensive dining establishments. If we did a comparison between the typical fast food menu of ten years ago and today, you'd realize that there have been significant changes. The menu has broadened its scope, and there are more healthy choices for people who monitor fat, cholesterol, sugar, and sodium intake. Evidence indicates that this trend will continue to reflect consumer demand. So, consumers, continue to demand healthier choices!

In fact, the large chains have spent millions convincing the nutrition-conscious American that they start off with healthy foods, such as 100 percent pure beef, or products from nationally recognized distributors. The problem does not really lie with the healthiness or the quality of the original products. The downfall of fast foods is the end products. Often, menu choices are calorie-, fat-, and sodium-dense due to the preparation methods used.

Several of the internationally known companies completely expose themselves by providing, on request, ingredient and nutrition information. As a consumer, you can have at your fingertips the sodium, fat, and cholesterol content – and more – of many fast foods. Many companies also provide diabetes exchange information for their foods. Consumers are encouraged to call or write for this information. The addresses and numbers of several large chains are listed at the end of this chapter in "For Further Information."

However, these efforts to serve a few healthier foods does not by any means suggest that fast foods are suddenly healthier. There are still many nutritional disasters lurking in the listings of available items. The companies continue to spend big bucks trying to derive more market share by developing many unhealthy items. For instance, in the recent past we've seen many of the big chains add fried chicken pieces to their compendium of food items. One company was recently advertising a new mouth-watering taste treat—a double hamburger layered with three different types of cheese. Obviously, this item isn't high on the list of healthy selections.

It might be surprising to some but it's possible to navigate around the menu listings and sit down with a relatively healthy fast food meal. Certainly, many unhealthy food selections bombard you at the door, and getting seated with only healthy food choices may be the biggest challenge. Holding your nose and closing your eyes may make it a bit difficult to order and get to your table.

The reality is that fast food restaurants, featuring everything from hamburgers to fish or pizza, abound in our cities and along our highways. There are presently over 8,000 McDonald's and 5,000 Kentucky Fried Chicken outlets. Those are just two of the many international chains and local spots. The list gets longer and longer as the demand for fast food remains strong.

Most people will, at least on occasion, swing by one of the many fast food restaurants. For the most part, the meals are quick, a known entity, accessible, and relatively inexpensive (though you no longer get change back from your dollar bill). So, once again, the art of picking and choosing the healthier menu listings is your best weapon for surviving a fast food meal.

A wide variety of fast food restaurants are seen today. It used to be that fast foods would simply conjure up images of hamburgers or fried chicken. Today, most of the popular ethnic foods are featured at fast food stops across the country. Pizza, eggroll, and tacos are all available at ethnically specific fast food stops.

Seafood, salads, and roast beef are found at yet other fast food outlets. This chapter will focus on the foods found at America's most popular fast food restaurants. Many of the other widely available fast foods are reviewed in other chapters. For instance, you'll find pizza discussed in Chapter 7, "Healthier Eating Out: Italian Style," fast food breakfasts reviewed in Chapter 17 on breakfasts and brunches, and submarine sandwiches in Chapter 16, which is a review of healthier eating out at lunchtime.

What to consider before ordering

Fast foods have nutrition pitfalls. For the most part, their standard fare is higher in fat, saturated fat, and sodium and lower in carbohydrate than we're being encouraged to consume. In addition, the protein selections are often red meat—the hamburger—or deep-fried chicken or fish that comes laden with fat. The favorite carbohydrate—potatoes—are drenched in fat and become a high-calorie starch.

Vegetables are often hard to find. You don't see much that's green and crunchy in an order consisting of a burger, fries, and shake. However, more salads and a few pieces of broccoli are seen now on some fast food menus. Lower fat and skim milk is now more available. Fruit, other than fruit juice, is one food group that is not represented at all. Some people might try to pass off the deep-fat-fried fruit pies as a fruit serving, but dietitians would be hard pressed to buy that one.

The major villain once again is fat. It is so easy to quickly eat a meal that is over 50 percent fat. Consider a few examples: a six-pack of chicken pieces and small order of French fries; a single cheeseburger and apple fruit pie; or a fried fish sandwich with a side of coleslaw. You also need to be aware of the type as well as the amount of fat you consume; are you eating saturated, monounsaturated, or polyunsaturated fat?

The biggest problem is that the great majority of fast foods are fried and therefore incorporate lots of fat and calories. They start out with chicken, fish, potatoes, all foods we're encouraged to eat, but then cook these foods in six inches of grease. So even if foods sound healthy, think about the preparation method used. It's best to avoid or minimize the fried foods. For example, if you want French fries, offset them with a no-frills hamburger, or if you want chicken pieces, complement that order with a side salad or baked potato. Obviously, if you avoid all fried foods, you'll be better off, but that is not easily accomplished.

Beyond simply calculating the added calories from fried foods, there should be concern about the types of fat you are consuming. Some recent criticism of fast foods has been focused on the unhealthiness of the fat used in food preparation. If you eat fried foods, it's best to have them fried in the healthier fats, mono and polyunsaturates. Unfortunately, not all of the fast food products are fried in the healthier fats. Due to the taste that America has grown to love, many French fries are still cooked in a combination of animal and vegetable shortening. The animal shortening is most often beef in origin. Note from the "Nutrition Information on Selected Fast Foods" at the end of this chapter that there is cholesterol in French fries. The cholesterol is not in the potato; it's coming from the beef fat in which the potatoes are fried.

From information provided by several of the large chains, it's apparent that many other fried foods are now fried in 100 percent vegetable shortening. The oils found in these shortenings are usually the mainly polyunsaturated soybean and cottonseed oils. They might be hydrogenated or partially hydrogenated, which does make them a bit more saturated. However, the good news is that they don't contain cholesterol because these oils are non-animal based in origin. If you frequent a particular national chain and are curious about what fats they use, simply write to the company for detailed information.

Beyond simply fried foods, there are other ways to pick up fast food fats. Consider the frequent additions to hamburgers—cheese, bacon, special sauces, or mayonnaise. These are all just about 100 percent fat. In addition, even though there are some healthier food choices, such as the salad bars, pre-packaged salads, and baked potatoes, these healthy foods often get laden with fats and become "not-so-healthy" foods. Consider the pre-packaged salad topped with chicken that has a low 107 calories but comes with a two-ounce package of Italian dressing that adds a couple of hundred more calories. Or be aware that the baked potato's calories will double when topped off with a combination of cheese sauce, bacon bits, and/or sour cream—all fat-dense foods.

A positive aspect of the healthier food choices, such as salads or baked potatoes, is that you can control what's added. You can significantly impact fat intake by avoiding the unhealthy additions. See the chart at the end of this chapter entitled "Little Changes Add Up to a Big Nutrition Difference." It provides examples of how making simple changes can create healthier fast food meals.

The high sodium content of fast food meals is another nutrition pitfall. The sodium needle rises as foods are coated in salty batters or as pickles, special sauces, cheese, bacon, salad dressings, and salt are added in food preparation. Consider some examples. Six chicken nuggets, a quarter-pound hamburger, and a roast beef sandwich all have in the range of 500–700 milligrams of sodium. Interestingly, the French fries often are blamed for adding lots of sodium, but they seem to ring in at a bit over 100 milligrams for a small order. It would not be unusual for a fast food meal to rise quickly to 1,000–2,000 milligrams of sodium. Observe the nutrition information table at the end of the chapter, which provides some sodium values for familiar foods.

Common sense tells you that to keep sodium down you must minimize the high-sodium ingredients. Avoid those foods mentioned that raise sodium content. Consider the salad: if you use vinegar, lemon juice, or simply one-half of the package of dressing, your sodium intake is drastically reduced. Needless to say, you're better off with plainer hamburgers—without the cheese, special sauces, bacon, or pickles. These changes will reduce fat content while also lowering sodium intake.

Managing the menu

Practicing the art of preplanning is helpful and actually easier to do in a fast food restaurant than in many other establishments. For the most part, you don't need to read through the menu; you know what's available. Whether you're in California, Indiana, or Connecticut, the menu, for the most part, reads the same. So the best practice is to firmly decide what you will have before walking through the doors. If you vacillate, you might be tormented by the smells and quickly persuaded to order unwisely. If you have a willing dining partner, give them your order prior to walking in, and go sit down. That way, you don't have to look at the menu board or all the foods people have on their trays.

Special requests are difficult though not impossible. If you remember back a few years, Burger King's slogan was "special orders don't upset us." One of their ad campaigns continues to say "have it your way," and, in fact, their nutrition information suggests making special requests, such as leaving the pickles off or having no salt added to your French fries as ways to reduce sodium intake. The biggest problem with making special requests in a fast food restaurant is that you might have to wait and therefore defeat the purpose of eating fast food. I recall once requesting that mustard be substituted for the usual mayonnaise on a ham sandwich. This request led to a long wait. Wiping the mayonnaise off and adding the mustard myself would have been much quicker. So weigh the advantages and disadvantages, determine the difficulty of your request, and count the people standing in line in back of you.

It's important to monitor your pace of eating. Granted, getting the job of eating done quickly is the main reason for going to fast food stops. And certainly the environment in a fast food restaurant fosters a quickened pace of eating. Remember, nevertheless, to eat slowly; take at least 15–20 minutes. Drive-thru windows are not recommended. There is nothing positive about this style of eating. You tend to eat very quickly, hardly tasting your food, and you might be driving while you're eating, which is both unhealthy and dangerous. It's important to take a few minutes out to eat. This does take some preplanning.

Portion control, one of the basic skills of healthy dining out, is a bit easier in fast food places compared with more pricey restaurants. First, the portions, as long as you order smartly, are relatively small. A single hamburger has between two and three ounces of meat, hardly a large portion. The salads, chicken nuggets, and fish and beef sandwiches also come in reasonable portions. There is no waiting to eat, with bread and butter or other munchies on the table. There are no appetizers to contemplate or to watch others gorge on while you are waiting for the main course. Also, dessert receives little attention. Turn these characteristics to your own benefit in controlling portions and calories consumed.

To control portions further and eat healthier, practice useful ordering. Avoid items containing such words as jumbo, super, double, triple, extra large, and big. These orders will lead you to larger-than-necessary portions. Stick with the smaller sizes; look for cues such as small, junior, or single.

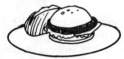

Typical Menu: Fast Food Style

There are many different fast food restaurants and more and more foods from which to choose. In this chapter most of the commonly available foods from nationally recognized chains are reviewed. The tables at the end of the chapter provide nutrient information for a representative sampling of various fast foods. If further nutrition information on a particular chain is desired, it is suggested that you contact the company.

Remember, too, that fast food breakfasts are discussed in Chapter 17, pizza in Chapter 7, and submarine sandwiches in Chapter 16.

Hamburgers	**There has** been lots of negative publicity about the contents of fast food hamburger patties. The large hamburger chains all state that they use 100 percent beef. They also typically add that it is United States Department of Agriculture (USDA) inspected meat. Another concern has been how the patties are prepared. Certainly, it is advantageous to broil beef because you lose fat in the cooking process.

It's fair to say that as the size of the hamburger and number of patties increase, so do the calories and fat. The small hamburger contains about two ounces of meat, the quarter-pound hamburgers have about three ounces cooked, and the doubles and triples have upwards of four ounces of meat. That does not even count the frequently added cheese, which adds protein, fat, and calories. Everyone remembers the commercial that aired several years ago with the slogan, "Where's the beef?" That was Wendy's commercial in which they bragged about their bigger hamburger patty. Healthwise, you are better off if you have to ask the question, "Where's the beef?" If you have a hard time finding the beef, it means you're likely consuming less saturated fat and cholesterol, at least from the hamburger.

It's also fair to say that as the number of additional ingredients increases, so do the calories and fat. The frequent additions to hamburgers are cheese, special sauces (usually mayonnaise based), bacon, pickles, onions, lettuce, tomatoes, mustard, and catsup. The last six are perfectly fine. They will significantly increase the flavor of the hamburger. The others will add taste but also add unhealthy ingredients. Compare the difference between a plain hamburger at Burger King with 275 calories, 39 percent of which are fat, to their bacon double cheeseburger, with 510 calories, 55 percent from fat. If you've got the calories to spare, it's definitely better to order two simple hamburgers rather than one with lots of meat and loaded with many high-fat ingredients.

Roast Beef Sandwiches There are a few chains specializing in sliced roast beef sandwiches. These might be a good change from the usual hamburger, both tastewise and for improved nutrition. Stick with the regular or junior-size sandwich. The roast beef sandwich is a bit lower in fat, cholesterol, and sodium than some of the larger hamburger choices. As with hamburgers, it's best to avoid the extras, such as cheese sauces.

Chicken Sandwiches

These sandwiches have a good healthy sound, but they are virtually always fried, so you get way more than just chicken. The sizes vary quite a bit from restaurant to restaurant. One benefit to the chicken sandwich is that it's slightly lower in saturated fat and cholesterol than moderate-size hamburgers. It seems that most places use 100 percent vegetable shortening to fry these items. Certainly, if the cheese and mayonnaise-based sauces are avoided, this is not a bad choice along with a salad or baked potato. With health consciousness in mind, several chains are introducing a grilled chicken sandwich. This will likely be a better alternative to the fried variety, but beware of the "special sauces."

Chicken Pieces

These were introduced first by McDonald's as Chicken McNuggets, and many chains have followed suit with their own versions. No matter whose version it is, however, these items are battered and fried, so the majority of calories come from fat. However, the Chicken Tenders served by Burger King and Chicken Strips served by Jack-In-The-Box are lower in fat and calories than several competitive products. These chicken pieces are available in varying portions. The smallest order, usually six pieces, is advised.

Chicken nuggets are served with a choice of three to four sauces, most of which have a sugary base—barbecue, mustard, sweet-and-sour, and honey. People who have diabetes should be aware that a two-ounce package of sauce can be considered a fruit exchange, but it's best to keep the quantity used to a minimum. Again, try to complement the chicken pieces with a low-fat and low-calorie side selection such as a tossed salad or baked potato filled with broccoli, hold the cheese.

Fried Chicken

There are several chains specializing in serving fried chicken to the masses. Kentucky Fried Chicken, or KFC to some, Church's, and Popeyes are a few of the larger chains. Generally speaking, there is very little to redeem these fast food spots. Even the coleslaw at some of them is over 50 percent fat. If you choose fried chicken, you are best off with the breast portion. Obviously, the fat and calories are decreased significantly by taking off the skin and breading. The crispier versions seem to add more fat and calories. If you eat fried chicken, try to set a limit of one piece, and complement it with mashed potatoes (no gravy) or corn on the cob rather than French fries, onion rings, or coleslaw. In a recent phone conversation from a public relations representative of Kentucky Fried Chicken, I was told that they are test marketing a grilled chicken breast. If this product becomes available, it might be a more nutritious offering.

Fried Seafood

Fried seafood is basically in the same class as fried chicken. The nutritious seafood is battered and fried, resulting in unhealthier and high-sodium food. There are several large chains around the country offering fast seafood: Long John Silver's and Captain D's are just two.

The products range from simple fried fish fillets to fried shrimp, oysters, and scallops. These items are often served with two more high-fat, high-calorie foods—French fries and creamy coleslaw. Long John Silver's does offer some broiled fish items, which are served with healthier side choices—rice pilaf, vegetable, side salad, or a dinner roll. Several of their seafood salads are also healthier choices.

Fried Fish Sandwiches

One of the early selections to follow hamburgers in the large chains was the fried fish fillet sandwich. Unfortunately, here is another good food destroyed by dunking it into vegetable shortening, adding mayonnaise-based sauces, and sometimes increasing saturated fat with cheese. If these are eaten, at least request that no extra sauce is used and order it without cheese. In general, there are better choices.

French Fries

It's probably more the exception than the rule when an order of French fries doesn't accessorize the fast food meal. Actually, considered on their own French fries are not that bad; the sodium content is low, there is minimal cholesterol (which comes from the frying medium), and the potato itself, though invaded by fat, does offer some nutrition. The problem is that the French fries accompany an already high-fat meal. If you order French fries, at least stick with a small order or consider sharing a large order with your fast food pal.

Baked Potatoes

In order to introduce an item that is a bit healthier to the cadre of choices, several chains now offer baked potatoes. Once again, we start off with one of the best nutritional bets, a potato, but we find a multitude of ways to increase the fat and calories by stuffing it with cheese, bacon, sour cream, chili, or a combination of several. The two fillers that are wise choices, broccoli and chives, are usually found in combination with cheese and sour cream. All in all, the baked potato stuffed with broccoli and cheese, or chili and cheese, is a bit wiser food choice. You might find them more filling than a small hamburger and fries. Observe the Low Calorie/Low Fat meals in the Model Meals section below.

Salads

The salads have been a welcomed food addition to the fast food menu. Several restaurant chains have introduced a salad bar while others have gone the pre-packaged salad route. These salads—tossed, chicken, chef, seafood, pasta, and others—are nutritious food choices either as a complete meal or to complement other selections.

The biggest problem with all of the salads is the dressing. The regular salad dressing, whether it's blue cheese, Thousand Island, or others, packs on another 100 or so calories, mostly from fat. Dressings also drastically raise the sodium content of a salad. Fast food restaurants use a two-ounce package. They say market research shows this is the volume desired by customers. You can reduce the calorie intake of salads by using a minimum of regular dressing, ordering the reduced-calorie variety, or just using vinegar or lemon juice. Several salads, such as the pasta salad and seafood salad, can be enjoyed without anything added. If you're closely monitoring sodium, it's worth noting that lower-calorie salad dressings are often higher in sodium than the regular varieties.

Several of the large chains continue to offer a salad bar. For more information on how to choose wisely at salad bars, refer to Chapter 15.

Beverages   There are numerous recommended beverage selections in fast food restaurants for the health-conscious consumer. Over the last ten years, more places stock low-fat and/or skim milk. Skim milk is the better choice if it's available. Fruit juice is available in some places. It's most often orange juice, which is a fine choice. Be careful that you are not ordering a fruit drink that is mainly sugar and water. For non-caloric beverages, one can choose from low-calorie carbonated drinks, hot coffee or tea, and iced tea. It's best to avoid the shakes. These usually add a few hundred calories and lots of fat. For further information on beverages, see Chapter 19.

In conclusion, here are some general words of caution about fitting fast food stops into your repertory of restaurant selections: 1) frequent these places sparingly; 2) carefully choose the items you will eat prior to putting your foot in the door; 3) balance a fast food meal by closely monitoring food choices the rest of the day.

Now that you've seen what may be available at fast food restaurants, look over the following "Model Meals" for suggestions on how to order to achieve specific nutritional goals. Models are numbered one to five for quick reference, and each is followed by an "Estimated Nutrient Evaluation" that analyzes the content of that meal.

May I Take Your Order

Healthy	30% Calories as fat
Daily	20% Calories as protein
Eating	50% Calories as carbohydrate
Goals	300 mg/day Cholesterol
	3000 mg/day Sodium

---

❶

Low Calorie/	**Baked potato** with chili and
Low Fat	cheese
Model Meal	*Quantity:* 1
	Exchanges: 1½ meat (med.); 2 fat; 4 starch
	Low-calorie carbonated beverage
	Quantity: unlimited
	Exchanges: free

Estimated	481 calories
Nutrient	35% calories as fat
Evaluation	19% calories as protein
	46% calories as carbohydrate
	31 mg cholesterol
	701 mg sodium

---

❶

Low Calorie/	**Hamburger,** single, with
Low Fat	condiments
Model Meal	*Quantity:* 1
	Exchanges: 2 meat (med.); 2 starch
	French fries
	Quantity: small order
	Exchanges: 2 fat; 1½ starch
	Iced tea, unsweetened (or sugar sub.)
	Quantity: unlimited
	Exchanges: free

Estimated Nutrient Evaluation	512 calories
	40% calories as fat
	13% calories as protein
	47% calories as carbohydrate
	47 mg cholesterol
	507 mg sodium

❷
Low Calorie/ Low Cholesterol Model Meal

Tossed salad with chicken (dressing on the side)
Quantity: 1 order
Oriental dressing (on the side)
Quantity: ½ pkg
Low-fat milk (skim preferable)
Quantity: 8 oz

Estimated Nutrient Evaluation	279 calories
	23% calories as fat
	37% calories as protein
	40% calories as carbohydrate
	90 mg cholesterol
	844 mg sodium

❸
Higher Calorie/Low Fat Model Meal

Chicken pieces
Quantity: 6 pieces
Exchanges: 2 meat (med.); 2 fat
Baked potato with broccoli and cheese
Quantity: 1
Exchanges: 4 fat; 1 vegetable; 3 starch
Orange juice
Quantity: 8 oz
Exchanges: 2 fruit

Estimated Nutrient Evaluation	804 calories
	42% calories as fat
	15% calories as protein
	43% calories as carbohydrate
	82 mg cholesterol
	1028 mg sodium

❹

Higher Calorie/Low Cholesterol Model Meal	**Hamburger,** with condiments *Quantity:* quarter-pound **French fries** *Quantity:* small order **Tossed salad** (dressing on the side) *Quantity:* 1 order **Reduced-calorie Italian dressing** (on the side) *Quantity:* ½ pkg **Low-fat milk** (skim preferable) *Quantity:* 8 oz
Estimated Nutrient Evaluation	837 calories 45% calories as fat 16% calories as protein 39% calories as protein 110 mg cholesterol 1373 mg sodium (990 mg without salad dressing)

❺

Low Sodium Model Meal	**Roast beef sandwich** *Quantity:* 1 regular **French fries** *Quantity:* small order **Tossed salad** (dressing on the side) *Quantity:* 1 order **Vinegar or lemon dressing** (on the side) *Quantity:* unlimited **Coffee or tea** *Quantity:* unlimited
Estimated Nutrient Evaluation	597 calories 37% calories as fat 18% calories as protein 45% calories as carbohydrate 63 mg cholesterol 825 mg sodium

*Little changes add up to a big nutrition difference**

CHANGE THIS ORDER:

	Total Cals	Fat (grams)	% Cals as fat	% Cals as carbo-hydrate	% Cals as protein	Sod-ium	Choles-terol
Quarter-pound hamburger with cheese and sauces	570	35	55	27	18	979	110
French fries, large	390	20	46	48	6	176	20
Cola beverage, regular	159	0	0	100	0	5	0
Totals	1019	55	34	58	8	1160	130

TO:

Regular hamburger without cheese and sauces	322	17	47	36	18	486	86
Baked potato	250	2	7	83	10	60	0
Tossed salad	42	0	0	64	56	23	0
Reduced-calorie dressing	50	4	70	30	0	360	0
Low-calorie beverage	1	0	0	0	0	10	0
Totals	655	23	31	55	14	939	86

CHANGE THIS ORDER:

Chicken specialty sandwich	688	40	52	33	15	1423	75
French fries, large	390	20	46	48	6	176	20
Chocolate shake	320	12	34	57	9	202	37
Totals	1398	72	42	44	14	1801	132

TO:

Chicken pieces	204	10	43	19	38	636	62
Baked potato with broccoli and cheese	541	22	37	53	10	475	20
Low-calorie beverage	1	0	0	0	0	10	0
Totals	746	32	40	36	24	1121	82

Nutrition information on selected fast foods* (see Abbreviations Key on page 247)

FOOD	Total Cals	Fat (grams)	% Cals as fat	% Cals as carbo-hydrate	% Cals as protein	Sod-ium mg	Choles-terol, mg
Hamburgers							
Hamburger, single (BK)	275	12	38	41	21	509	37
Cheeseburger, single (McD)	318	16	45	35	20	743	41
Hamburger, single (W)	350	16	41	31	28	360	75
Whopper Jr., no cheese (BK)	322	17	47	36	18	486	41
Quarter-Pounder with cheese (McD)	525	32	54	23	23	1220	107
Bacon double cheese-burger (W)	510	31	54	21	25	728	112
Whopper with cheese (BK)	711	43	55	27	18	1164	113
Roast Beef Sandwiches							
Roast beef sandwich (A)	353	15	38	37	25	590	52
Roast beef sandwich with cheese (A)	490	21	39	51	24	1520	77
Chicken Sandwiches							
Chicken Specialty sandwich (BK)	688	40	52	33	15	1423	66
Chicken sandwich (W)	320	10	29	39	32	500	60
Grilled chicken fillet (JB)	408	17	37	32	31	1130	64
Chicken breast fillet with cheese (DQ)	661	38	52	29	19	921	87
Chicken Pieces							
Chicken Tenders, 6 (BK)	204	10	43	19	38	636	47
Chicken Strips, 4 (JB)	349	14	36	32	33	748	68
Chicken McNuggets, 6 (McD)	323	20	56	19	25	512	63
Kentucky Nuggets, 6 (KFC)	276	17	55	20	25	840	62

Nutrition information on selected fast foods (continued)

FOOD	Total Cals	Fat (grams)	% Cals as fat	% Cals as carbo- hydrate	% Cals as protein	Sod- ium mg	Choles- terol, mg
Sauces (2 tbsp)							
Hot mustard (McD)	63	2	29	67	4	259	3
Barbecue (KFC)	35	0	0	80	0	450	0
Sweet-and-sour (W)	45	0	0	97	0	55	0
Fried Chicken							
Center breast, Original (KFC)	257	14	49	11	40	532	74
Center breast, Extra Crispy (KFC)	353	21	54	16	30	842	74
Thigh, Original (KFC)	278	19	62	12	26	517	83
Thigh, Extra Crispy (KFC)	371	26	63	16	21	766	83
Fried Seafood							
Fish fillets (2) with fries (LJS)	651	36	50	33	17	1352	62
Shrimp (6) with fries and coleslaw (LJS)	711	45	57	34	9	1297	215
Baked fish dinner, coleslaw, mixed vegetables (LJS)	387	19	44	20	36	1298	75
Fried Fish Sandwiches							
Fried fish sandwich (LJS)	406	15	34	41	25	1029	55
Filet-O-Fish (McD)	435	26	54	33	13	799	47
Whaler (BK)	488	27	49	36	15	592	77
French Fries, small							
French fries (McD)	220	12	48	47	5	109	9
French fries (W)	310	15	45	49	6	105	15
French fries (DQ)	200	10	45	50	5	114	10
Baked Potatoes							
Baked potato (W)	250	2	7	83	10	60	0
Baked potato with cheese and broccoli (A)	541	22	37	53	10	475	20
Baked potato with chili and cheese (W)	510	20	34	49	17	610	22

Nutrition information on selected fast foods (continued)

Food	Total Cals	Fat (grams)	% Cals as fat	% Cals as carbo- hydrate	% Cals as protein	Sod- ium mg	Choles- terol, mg
Salads, no dressing							
Tossed salad (A)	44	0	0	63	27	23	0
Salad with chicken (USDA)	105	2	19	15	66	209	72
Chef salad (USDA)	267	16	54	7	39	744	139
Mexican salad (JB)	442	31	46	27	26	1500	89
Ocean salad (LJS)	222	8	32	17	51	983	150
Salad Dressing, 2 oz							
Blue cheese (BK)	156	16	92	5	3	309	22
Thousand Island (W)	140	14	90	10	0	230	10
Lite Italian (W)	50	4	70	30	0	360	0

Abbreviation Key:

A   Arby's
BK   Burger King
DQ   Dairy Queen
JB   Jack-In-The-Box
KFC   Kentucky Fried Chicken
LJS   Long John Silver's
McD   McDonald's
USDA United States Department of Agriculture information used when not available from specific company
W   Wendy's

*References used throughout chapter for nutrition evaluation:

1. "Composition of Foods: Fast Foods," United States Department of Agriculture Human Nutrition Information Service, *Agricultural Handbook 8-21,* 1988.
2. Specific company information utilized when available. Most currently available information utilized, 1986–present.
+3. Franz, M. J., *Fast Food Facts, Nutritive and Exchange Values for Fast Food Restaurants,* 1987, Diabetes Center, Inc., P.O. Box 739, Wayzata, MN 55391.

For further information

Arby's
Suite 700
3495 Piedmont Rd.
Atlanta, GA 30305

800-2-ADVISE

Burger King
Corporation
Consumer Relations,
Mail Station 1490
P.O. Box 520783,
General Mail Facility
Miami, FL 33152

305-378-7320

Home Economist
International Dairy
Queen, Inc.
P.O. Box 35286
Minneapolis, MN 55435

612-830-0200

Kentucky Fried Chicken
Public Affairs Dept.
P.O. Box 32070
Louisville, KY 40232

502-456-8300

Long John Silver's
Nutrition Dept.
Jerrico, Inc.
P.O. Box 11988
Lexington, KY 40579

606-268-2000

McDonald's Nutrition
Information Center
Customer Relations
McDonald's Plaza
Oakbrook, IL 60521

312-575-FOOD

Wendy's International,
Inc.
Consumer Affairs Dept.
P.O. Box 256
Dublin, OH 43017

614-764-6800

15

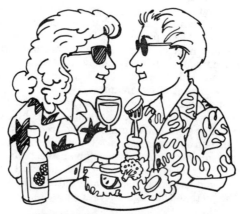

Healthier eating out
Salad Bar Style

Y ou guys go have your burgers and fries, it's the salad bar for me. I'm watching my waistline." How many times have you heard this virtuous statement echoed in the employee cafeteria or a local fast food haven? Unfortunately, the well intended "healthy" trip, or trips, to an all-you-can-eat salad bar often results in a shockingly high-fat and high-calorie meal.

The word "salad" does bring to mind visions of lettuce, spinach, tomatoes, and peppers in a rainbow of colors. All of these salad ingredients offer a lot of bulk, vitamins, minerals, and—best news of all—very few calories. However, in and among these healthy salad bar "regulars" lurks the pasta salad, potato salad, marinated vegetables, pepperoni, cheeses, and other high-fat foods that also boost calories way up. Lastly, to add insult to injury, the salad is topped off with dressing, often containing upward of 60 or 70 calories per tablespoon. So, under the guise of a "healthy" food choice, the salad bar, if not approached cautiously, can result in a very high-fat and high-calorie meal.

However, when approached with a plan in mind, more knowledge about wise and unwise food selections, and lots of self-discipline, the salad bar can be a nutritionally complete lunch or dinner. Salad bars are convenient, relatively inexpensive, quick, and easy. They can fill the bill for a meal eaten out or a take-out meal brought home. Salad bars are especially handy and refreshing in the warm weather–when preparing a meal is particularly unappetizing and you're tempted to just sit down with the cheese and crackers or pint of ice cream.

Having a salad bar available as part of your meal can be quite helpful in the pursuit of healthier eating out. The salad can be quite filling. And if you partially fill up on low-calorie raw vegetables, it's easier to eat a smaller portion of the main entree. If you can immediately make your trip to the salad bar, it's easier to avoid the bread basket and butter. The salad also helps take the edge off your appetite.

The vast array of salad options

Today, salad bars are found in many types of eating spots, from fast food stops to family restaurants and American steakhouses. Salad bars are also becoming more and more familiar sights in our large supermarkets. By having salad bars available, supermarkets capture on-the-run lunch and dinner traffic as well as the no-time-to-cut-everything-up crowd. Locally, in Boston, several large supermarkets have well-stocked salad bars complete with many very fresh ingredients.

Salad bars are also frequently seen in employee cafeterias at hospitals, business complexes, and even in school cafeterias. It's common to pay by the ounce at these salad bars. At family restaurants and steakhouses, the salad can be the whole meal or simply an adjunct. The fast food industry caught onto the salad bar trend in the early eighties, and most large chains offer some type of salad. Several operations such as Wendy's, Taco Bell, and Papa Gino's offer the make-your-own salad bars. A few chains, McDonald's, Jack-in-the-Box, and Burger King, for example, offer pre-packaged salads. They have a variety of selections and dressings from which to choose.

Americans can definitely claim the all-you-can-eat salad bar as our invention. The biggest problem with them is that you often eat what you consider your "money's worth." That frequently means you overeat. All-you-can-eat salad bars are certainly the perfect set up for a pig-out. And since it is under the guise of health—lots of vegetables—you can really fool yourself.

Practicing self-discipline at the salad bar

Those people who feel their will power, or, better stated, won't power, just doesn't hold up around a tempting salad bar, might best avoid them. In fact, some people might be better off choosing a hamburger, small order of French fries, and diet soda rather than risk overindulgence at the salad bar. If you are extremely hungry, being unleashed at the salad bar can be particularly disastrous.

There are a few strategies one may use to solve the problem of wavering self-discipline. If you have a sympathetic friend, you might be able to coerce him or her into going to the salad bar for you. You can specify your order at the table after surveying the salad bar. The willing friend exercises portion control and places just the items you should have on your plate.

Another suggestion is to go to the salad bar yourself, but use a smaller plate. Often times there are small and large plates or bowls available. If you use the smaller of the two, you can only put so much on it. This is portion control at its simplest level. Lastly, limit yourself to just one trip; don't even think about going back for seconds.

Those choosing fast food places for salads might want to stick with the pre-packaged variety. If you feel your self-control is limited at the all-you-can-eat salad bars, the pre-packaged salad might work better. These salads range from a low of 32 calories for a 1½-cup tossed salad with no dressing to a high of

380 calories for 1½ cups of tossed salad with the addition of pasta salad (not including dressing). (More nutrient evaluation of fast food salads may be found in Chapter 14, "Healthier Eating Out: Fast Food Style.") Self-control is, however, needed with the packet of salad dressing. In my estimation, the packets often contain enough for three salads. As dressing is a large contributor of calories, you are best off using the lower-calorie offerings and certainly not the whole package.

What to consider when approaching the salad bar

Before you even approach the salad bar, take a minute or two to do some preplanning, even if it's just on your walk from the parking lot or to the employee cafeteria. Think about how hungry you are. If hunger is about to get the better of you, remember, your eyes are probably bigger than your stomach. Rather than choosing with your eyes and taste buds, try to make decisions with your meal plan and health goals in mind. Think about what foods you really want, and in what quantity. If you are unfamiliar with a particular salad bar, or items are constantly changing, take a moment to survey the situation. Observe what is available prior to selecting.

Nutritionally speaking, salad bars can be great either as part of or as the entire meal. Offerings can be chosen to fit into a variety of different meal plans and health goals. They can give you plenty of carbohydrates along with lots of soluble fiber. Greens and vegetables assist in keeping the protein portion of your meal low and can, if you choose wisely, help keep fat, saturated fat, and cholesterol to a minimum.

From a sodium standpoint, salad bars can again range from great to disastrous. Vegetables are extremely low in sodium, but you can get into trouble with some of the salad mixtures—macaroni salad, coleslaw—or the ham, olives, pickles, and croutons. The best advice no matter what your nutritional goals is to load up on the veggies.

As you begin making your choices, start with the raw vegetables. These are usually placed at the beginning of the salad bar. Often, very low-calorie vegetables—lettuce, spinach, cucumbers, broccoli, celery, mushrooms, sprouts, and others—are available.

(See Table 1 at the end of this chapter, which delineates the best and the worst salad bar choices.) Vegetables provide plenty of crunch and volume with very few calories. Raw vegetables also give the visual image of having lots on your plate, but they weigh in lighter than many high-fat choices. Compare, for example, sliced cucumbers with pasta salad, or bean sprouts with chunks of cheddar cheese. If you're at a salad bar that charges by the ounce, you'll even end up with a few extra cents in your pocket by choosing the high-volume, low-calorie foods.

The next ingredients to be layered on your salad plate are the slightly higher calorie but still very healthy items such as beets, chick peas, tuna, and others. You'll find several vegetables that are a bit higher in calories but by all means still very nutritious: carrots, beets, and onions are among these selections.

There are usually several items on the salad bar that help you add more carbohydrate without adding much fat—green peas, chick peas (also known as garbanzo beans), and kidney beans are among them. Chick peas and kidney beans might also be found in three-bean salad, which makes a frequent appearance at salad bars. For the most part, three bean is one of the better mixed salads to choose because it contains practically no fat. People with diabetes might want to avoid it, however, because sugar is added to most three-bean salad mixes.

Croutons, crackers, pita pockets, and breads are often found at the salad bar. A few croutons are fine, although they might be high in sodium. You should particularly avoid homemade croutons in better restaurants as they often are the fat-drenched variety.

For those wishing to add some relatively low-calorie protein foods to their salad, here are several choices: plain tuna (not mixed into tuna salad), ham, egg, feta cheese, and cottage cheese (likely, it will not be low fat). Two of these—ham and feta cheese—are high in sodium. (See Table 3 below.) Obviously, tuna, chicken, and seafood salad add protein, but they also add lots of fat. Cheese and pepperoni contain more calories from fat than from protein, and pepperoni especially adds sodium.

The bigger the salad bar, the more salad mixtures are available such as pasta salads, marinated vegetable salads, and others. Some of these are smart choices, and others should be left in the serving bowl. Generally speaking, marinated beets, marinated mixed vegetables or mushrooms, three-bean salad, a vinegar-based coleslaw, and mixed fruit salad are fine. Small quantities (about ¼ cup) should be taken, especially by those closely monitoring calories, sugar, and sodium intake.

The magic to keeping the calorie count of your salad down (excluding the dressing) is to take little or none of the mayonnaise, sour cream, and oil-based salad-mixtures. The pasta or macaroni salad, potato salad, coleslaw, and tuna, chicken, or seafood salad will increase your calorie intake quickly. Another item seen on salad bars is fruit ambrosia. This usually is made with sour cream, syrup-packed fruits, and marshmallows; try to avoid it.

Another place to pick up some hidden fat calories and possibly sodium is from the salad bar "accessories". There, temptations include nuts, seeds, Chinese dried noodles, olives, and bacon bits. Granted, these are usually added in small quantities, but observe their surprisingly high calorie contribution from the table that follows.

The lowdown on salad dressings

By far the biggest culprit in adding abundant and hidden calories is the crowning touch—salad dressing. Though I've never seen a survey, through talking to many people over the years I'm convinced that America's two favorite salad dressings are blue cheese and Thousand Island. Of course, these are among the highest fat and highest calorie dressings. Regular salad dressing, the type most frequently found at salad bars, rings in at about 60–80 calories per tablespoon. That's a level tablespoon, not heaping. In addition to the calories, the creamy dressings that contain mayonnaise, sour cream, and/or cheese have additional saturated fat not to be found in soy, cottonseed, or olive-oil-based salad dressings.

On average, people use at least two to four tablespoons of dressing on a salad. The packets of dressing given out in several fast food restaurants contain four tablespoons of dressing. I remember questioning a McDonald's representative at an American Dietetic Association meeting about why in the world they package such a large quantity. She responded by saying that market research has shown that that is the average quantity used by most people. Four tablespoons may even be underestimating for a large salad-bar salad. Simple mathematics tell you that this can add up to around 300–400 calories just for the dressing! And those calories are practically all fat. Observe table 2, which presents "The Low Down on Salad Dressings."

Salad dressings even though used in minimal quantity can contribute lots of sodium. Average sodium values are also provided in the table, "The Low Down on Salad Dressings." Four tablespoons of either a regular or reduced-calorie dressing can provide in the range of 500 milligrams of sodium. That's just from the dressing. Some of the no-oil dressings are even higher in sodium. Think about simply using oil and vinegar, which contains next to no sodium.

By no means must you eat your salad without dressing. There are lots of healthy options. First, start by using less of your favorite dressing. Think about how much is usually left on the plate. Another option is to take half the amount of your favorite dressing and thin it with vinegar, lemon juice, or water. This cuts the calories (and also sodium) in half. From 400 to 200 is certainly a significant reduction. And believe it or not, using less dressing helps you enjoy the various tastes of the foods more.

These days it's common to find at least one reduced-calorie or "light" salad dressing. These dressings range from about 15–30 calories per tablespon. That's half or less than half the calories of regular dressing. Oil-free dressings are available in the supermarket in great abundance but are nowhere to be found at salad bars. These dressings range from 2–8 calories per tablespoon. Available to purchase in the supermarket especially for restaurant dining are individually packaged no-oil salad dressings. These are found in the special diet section. They are an expensive way to go, but they might be a big help.

Another option that some people choose is to carry a portion of their preferred salad dressing in a small plastic container. Obviously, this is easier for women than men. If you often use the salad bar at work and there is a refrigerator available, consider keeping your dressing of choice in the refrigerator, and bring it to the cafeteria with you. Best yet, keep a bottle of regular, raspberry, or balsamic vinegar on hand.

Salad Bar Style

Some people enjoy vinegar with a bit of alternative sweetener, for instance, Equal or Sweet 'n Low. For piquancy, lemon or lime wedges are often available, especially at restaurants that serve liquor.

If you have adequate self-discipline, a plan in mind, and some knowledge about what to select and what to avoid, a salad bar can be the health-conscious eater's paradise. Check on the tables and you'll see that a few small selection changes can really add up to a big difference in the health quotient of your salad. That can make the salad bar a welcome option in a variety of dining establishments—family restaurants, fast food stops, your employee cafeteria, and even the supermarket for a quick take-out lunch or dinner.

TABLE 1

From best to worst in salad bar choices

Low-Calorie Vegetables (approx. 25 calories/1 cup)	Higher-Calorie Vegetables (approx. 25 calories/½ cup)
broccoli	artichoke, canned
cabbage (red or green)	beets, canned
cauliflower	carrots, raw
celery	onions, raw (all types)
cucumbers	tomatoes, raw
endive	
lettuce (all types)	
peppers (all types)	
radishes	
sauerkraut*	
spinach	
sprouts (all types)	
summer squash, raw	
watercress	
zucchini, raw	

Starches (60–100 calories/½ cup)	Lean Protein (40–80 calories/oz.)	Higher-Fat Protein (100+ calories/oz.)
chick peas (garbanzo beans)	plain tuna	cheeses*
kidney beans	cottage cheese	pepperoni*
green peas	egg	
croutons (commercial)	ham*	
crackers (4–6)	feta cheese*	
bread (1 slice or 1 oz)		
pita pocket (½)		

Salad Bar Mixtures (35–50 calories/¼ cup)	Salad Bar Mixtures (50–80 calories/¼ cup)
marinated/pickled beets	tuna salad
marinated artichoke hearts	chicken salad
three-bean salad	seafood salad
marinated assorted vegetables	corn relish
marinated mushrooms	macaroni salad
pasta salad, oil based	potato salad
gelatin with fruit	fruit ambrosia
fruit salad	pasta salad, mayonnaise-based

TABLE 1

From best to worst in salad bar choices (continued)

Salad Bar "Accessories" (calories/tablespoon)	
pickles*	2-5
hot peppers	2-5
raisins	10
Chinese noodles	20
bacon bits (soy based)	27
sunflower seeds	47
olives, green or black*	50
peanuts	50
sesame seeds	52

*Items particularly high in sodium.

TABLE 2

*The lowdown on salad dressings**

	Cals/ tbsp	Fat/ grams	% cals fat	% saturated fat+	Sodium/ mg
Regular Dressings					
Blue cheese	77	8.0	94	19	22
French	67	6.4	86	23	213
Italian	69	7.1	93	14	116
Mayonnaise					
(soy and safflower)	99	11.0	100	11	78
Russian	76	7.8	92	14	113
Thousand Island	59	NA	85	16	109
Olive oil	119	13.5	100	13	0
Soybean and cottonseed oil	120	13.6	100	18	0
Low or Reduced-Calorie Dressings					
Blue cheese	27	<1*	30	NA	NA
French	22	.9	36	11	128
Italian	16	1.5	84	13	118
Russian	23	.7	27	14	141
Thousand Island	24	1.6	60	13	153
No-Oil Dressings					
Walden Farms Italian	9	<1*	30	NA	300
Wishbone Italian	6	0*	0	NA	210
Dressing Alternatives					
Vinegar (any type)	2	0	0	0	trace
Lemon or lime juice	4	0	0	0	0

*Reference used for this table is "Composition of Foods: Fats and Oils," United States Department of Agriculture Human Nutrition Information Service, *Agricultural Handbook 8-4*, 1979.

+There is minimal cholesterol in any of these products because they usually contain fats of non-animal origin. Dressings that contains eggs, egg yolk, cream, sour cream, cheese, or other animal-source items will contain small quantities of cholesterol.

*Information obtained from the product label.

NA Information not available.

TABLE 3

A few changes add up to a big difference at the salad bar
Note: *First 7 items are included in all 4 examples.*

Your Regular Salad	A Few Changes	A Few More	And One More
1 cup lettuce ¼ cup cucumbers ¼ cup peppers ¼ cup fresh mushrooms ⅛ cup alfalfa sprouts ⅛ cup shredded carrots ¼ cup green peas	(SAME)	(SAME)	(SAME)
¼ cup tuna salad 1 oz cheddar cheese 1 oz pepperoni ¼ cup potato salad ¼ cup macaroni salad 1 tbsp sunflower seeds	1 oz feta cheese 2 oz diced ham ¼ cup three-bean salad ¼ cup potato salad 2 tsp sunflower seeds	1 oz cottage cheese 2 oz tuna (plain) ¼ cup coleslaw ¼ cup sliced beets ¼ cup croutons	(SAME)
4 tbsp Thousand Island dressing	4 tbsp reduced-calorie Thousand Island dressing	2 tbsp reduced-calorie Thousand Island dressing and 3 tbsp vinegar	5 tbsp vinegar
Total calories 767	479	361	317
Grams of fat 60	25	8	5
% cals as fat 70	46	20	14
Sodium 1647 mg	1275 mg	958 mg	652 mg
Cholesterol 145 mg	52 mg	45 mg	41 mg

16

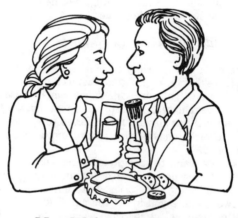

Healthier eating out
Luncheon Style

Surprisingly, lunch is the meal most frequently eaten away from home. The National Restaurant Association adds that over half of consumers eat lunch out at least once a week. Lunch is eaten out in a wide gamut of restaurants and for a variety of reasons. Where people eat lunch is dependent on several factors: time constraints, their budget, the purpose of the lunch, and the available restaurants.

If you're working, you have certain parameters for choosing a luncheon spot. If you have half an hour, obviously you won't venture very far. If you travel and eat lunch between appointments, you'll likely choose among the restaurants on your route that day. Those of you who work at home, are retired, or in other situations might have a bit more flexibility in determining luncheon spots.

Some people eat lunch daily in their work-site cafeteria, whereas others might venture out to a fast food joint, a mall eatery, or a local sandwich shop. Still others might find themselves out celebrating a fellow employee's birthday or retirement while some might be having an elaborate business lunch, integrating light cuisine with heavy negotiations. Whatever the situation, the skills and strategies of healthier eating out still play the key role.

The wide gamut of lunch spots

There's a wide variety of luncheon stops to talk about. We'll review some great menu choices for each type. There will also be "OK" suggestions. These are not the best choices, nutritionally speaking, but OK especially if you have a few calories to spare. The poorer choices, ones to steer away from, will also be mentioned.

The restaurants to be critiqued begin with sandwich shops—places where you can order sandwiches, soups, salads, and a few accessories. Next delicatessens are reviewed, where you know you can find lots of unhealthy menu selections such as chopped liver, hot pastrami, and a Reuben; but there are also healthy choices. Finally, submarine shops will be reviewed, followed by a brief discussion of what's available at the newer mall eateries. We'll also provide some strategies for dealing with the work-site cafeteria.

Obviously, there are many other categories of restaurants frequented for lunch. Several biggies are fast food stops, American cafes (serving hamburgers, salads, and sandwiches), pizza parlors, and quick ethnic eateries—Chinese, Mexican, and Middle Eastern. These and others are discussed in depth in other chapters of the book. The Table of Contents will assist you in locating the appropriate chapters.

What to consider before ordering

Lunch is a meal more likely to fall into the same routine than dinner. For lunch, people get caught in a groove and eat similar foods day after day, year after year. Most of us are more interested in planning for dinner, either at home or eating out. Unfortunately, the groove people frequently get caught in is a high-fat one, and they often don't realize it. For instance, many people tolerate a tuna salad, bologna, or salami sandwich rotation forever. They are simply on automatic pilot when ordering out or carrying lunch from home. The goal is simply to get the mission of eating lunch accomplished rather than worrying much about what is eaten. Often that sandwich is complemented with a bag of chips, order of French fries, or creamy coleslaw. Unknowingly, a high-fat lunch has been eaten.

Consider the example of the healthy-sounding tuna salad sandwich, served on whole-wheat bread spread with a mere three ounces of tuna, topped with lettuce and tomato, and served with a good size handful of chips on the side. Without even adding in the frequently ordered can of cola, the calories are up to about 600, with about 45 percent coming from fat. The calories would bounce up to about 750 with a regular soda. That's a chunk of calories for a quick, get-the-job-done lunch.

That's not even the worst of possible choices! Think about the submarine sandwiches that look like they go on forever, filled with Genoa salami, mortadella, and provolone cheese. Or think about the frequently ordered hot pastrami sandwich in a delicatessen, often served with potato salad or creamy coleslaw or both. Obviously, these examples show you that lots of damage can be done in the fat and calorie department when you're simply choosing a "quick and easy" lunch.

Once again, careful attention to foods high in fat is the first consideration when deciding what to order. If you're ordering a sandwich, think about choosing lean items and those not mixed with lots of mayonnaise. Be careful of added accessories—potato chips, French fries, coleslaw, and potato salad are all high-fat items. Think about asking for substitutes or ordering alternative side dishes such as a tossed salad, vinegar-based coleslaw, sliced tomatoes and lettuce, or a big pickle (if you can handle the sodium). If you want a crunchy addition of potato, corn, or tortilla chips, consider grabbing a bag of popcorn or pretzels as lower-fat alternatives. You still get the crunch but lots less fat.

Have a plan in mind—know what you will order before you go. More times than not, you've probably been at that establishment fairly often, so you know the offerings. If you use the work-site cafeteria, you know all too well what's available. Take advantage of eating where you work, but bring along the items that are unavailable, for example, a low-calorie salad dressing or fresh fruit. This strategy is also acceptable in most local sandwich shops and delicatessens, and you certainly can do it in the mall eateries.

Remember the basic principles of portion control. Even though it's lunch and you expect the portions to be smaller, they're still often larger than necessary, especially for the weight watchers. Think about sharing. Maybe one of you orders a sandwich and the other a Greek or garden salad. I bet you'd both end up with a perfect balance of vegetables, starches, and protein, with minimal fats and sodium. Or use the option sometimes provided of ordering soup and a half-sandwich or simply a half-sandwich with salad.

Be assertive; don't be dragged by friends or coworkers to places where you don't want to be. And don't be talked into ordering or sharing items you know it's best to avoid. Many people simply want a partner in crime and feel better if someone else is also eating greasy fries or indulging in a post-lunch ice cream cone.

In one of my weight control groups, one woman, who has lost about 40 pounds, discussed the fact that her coworkers can't wait for her to get "off" her diet so they can once again enjoy the fried onion rings they indulged in prior to her starting "that diet." We encouraged her to remind her coworkers that she will be watching her calories for a long time to come and, at most, a *shared* order of fried onion rings will be enjoyed on occasion.

SANDWICH SHOPS

There's a wide variety of sandwich shops to choose from when you're out doing errands or getting through a hectic workday. There are the local sandwich shops, or what might be called coffee shops. In some of these spots it's typical to see tuna or chicken salad, hamburgers, soups, and salad plates on the menu. In others the menu might read more like a combination coffee shop and delicatessen. Actually, some chains of ice cream stores double as places for a quick sandwich, for example, Swensen's and Friendly's.

There are also some newer sandwich shops and chains that, for lack of a better definition, we'll call "nouvelle" sandwich shops. You'll likely find sandwiches served on croissants or baguettes, and you'll have your choice of regular, Dijon, or Pommery mustard if desired. Usually soups and salads are also available. Generally speaking, these places offer healthier choices.

Best choices

Whatever the aura, food listings are often quite similar from one sandwich spot to the next. There are some great healthy choices on most of these menus. Don't shy away from sandwiches, thinking the bread is loaded with calories. Remember, it's what's between the slices that's the problem. So don't go taking off the top part of the roll or bread and just eating the insides and the bottom half. You're better off taking out and sharing the meat and eating all the bread.

There are usually various breads from which to choose. Often the listings include white, whole-wheat, light and dark rye, hard rolls, croissants, and Syrian pocket bread. If you can get a 100 percent whole-wheat bread, that's great, because you're picking up some insoluble fiber. The croissant is definitely a choice to avoid; it's loaded with fat. Syrian pocket, or pita bread, as it is often called, is a great choice, especially if you are closely watching calories.

The best sandwich fillers are turkey breast, sliced chicken, grilled chicken breast, roast beef, and ham. If you are on a very low sodium meal plan, ham might not be the right choice, but otherwise, on occasion, it's a fine alternative. Try to avoid the cheese, often layered on top. You've already got plenty of protein, and you don't need the fat and cholesterol from cheese. Request that the meat be topped with plenty of lettuce and tomato to expand the volume. Be careful to instruct the waitperson or preparer not to add butter, margarine, or mayonnaise to the bread. Think about using mustard, ketchup, or horseradish (if available) to moisten the bread and spice up the sandwich with very few calories and no fat.

OK Choices

Unfortunately, we often see the healthy choices of tuna, seafood sticks, crabmeat, and chicken combined with lots of mayonnaise. For this reason, these items, either in a sandwich or on a salad, aren't as good choices as the above. You might want to ask the wait-person if the tuna or chicken salad is very moist; if not, try it. But certainly request that no other mayonnaise be added to the bread.

Other OK choices in sandwich shops are the frequently found garden, Greek, and chef salads. Don't forget to ask for dressing on the side and a low-calorie one if it's available. On the chef salad, you might want to ask that the egg and/or cheese be left off. You might also want to request that more turkey or ham be substituted, but that's really not necessary as you'll already get plenty of protein. A bacon, lettuce, and tomato sandwich, as long as the mayonnaise is not slathered on, is actually not a bad choice on occasion. There are usually only two or three strips of bacon, and you should request that it be crisp. A small hamburger is also an OK choice. Try to get lettuce, tomato, and onion added to expand the volume with few calories.

There might be a few soup offerings that please your palate. Look for brothy-type soups such as chicken, beef, vegetable with noodles or rice, split pea, lentil, barley, or tomato. A cup of chili might even be available. Homemade soups are best because they'll have less sodium than canned ones. Avoid creamy soups, such as New England clam chowder, creamy broccoli, cream of mushroom, or cream of anything. Perhaps a cup of soup and salad will be on the menu, or a cup of soup and half a sandwich.

Worst choices

Sandwich shops definitely offer a few unhealthy choices worth avoiding. Paradoxically, the name "diet plate" should be a signal to look in another direction. These plates arrived on the scene when protein was "in" and breads were "out." The diet plate usually has a big hamburger and a hefty scoop of cottage cheese; both contribute mostly protein. There's little carbohydrate to be found, other than the typical peach half and maybe a few crackers. But there's lots of fat, saturated at that, from the protein.

In addition, it's best to avoid egg salad, cheeseburgers, grilled cheese, or cheese sandwiches. Also watch out for the melts—tuna melt is probably most well known, but cheese is often found melted over chicken salad, seafood salad, and cold cuts. Steer clear of combination sandwiches that pack on the meats and sometimes cheeses—roast beef and turkey, ham and turkey, or ham, turkey, and Swiss. These combo sandwiches end up with about six ounces of meat, more protein than most of us need for the entire day. Club sandwiches are also best avoided because of the large portion.

DELICATESSENS

Although the word "kosher" is usually used in association with delis, there are actually very few truly kosher delicatessens. Truly kosher means the establishment purchases, prepares, and serves foods according to the rules of *kashrut* (Jewish dietary laws). There are many kosher-style delicatessens and even more delicatessens that really, by definition, are sandwich shops.

The first foods that come to mind when you hear the frequently used abbreviation "deli" are knockwurst, hot pastrami, chopped liver, and bagels spread thickly with cream cheese and topped with lox (smoked salmon). These commonly served foods are high in fat and often sodium. A delicatessen might not be the best restaurant choice for lunch, or any meal at that, but if your arm is twisted and you find yourself sitting in one of the cozy booths, there are some fine menu choices. There are, sadly, more tempting treats with which to avoid eye contact.

Best Choices

Beef brisket, turkey breast, smoked turkey, lean roast beef—all are fine choices. In many delis you'll find extra-lean corned beef and pastrami. The biggest problem is that the sandwiches are loaded with meat. The bread hardly balances on top of the pile of thinly sliced meat. A great idea for portion control is to have one person order the sandwich and the other request two slices of bread or a roll. Split the portion of meat, and you'll each have a reasonable quantity. Or if there are no willing dining partners, order a half-sandwich with an extra slice of bread. Delis often have half-sandwiches listed on the menu.

OK Choices

Some other relatively nutritious choices are tuna salad, chicken salad, and chopped herring. These are usually available as a sandwich or salad plate. Again, the portions are large and splitting a sandwich is a great idea. Prior to ordering the salad plate, determine if it comes with an additional scoop of creamy coleslaw and/or potato salad. If it does, ask if you can substitute crackers, bread, or a roll.

A chef salad, with substitutions if needed; a bagel with cream cheese on the side (use a small amount); a bowl of brothy soup; borscht (beet soup), hold the sour cream; and the fresh fruit plate with cottage cheese are all sensible alternatives.

The frequently found accompaniments in a delicatessen can range from nutritional disaster, such as potato salad, to good choices, such as vinegar-based coleslaw or sauerkraut (as long as you can handle the sodium). Try to avoid the mayonnaise-based salads and go for the tossed salad, sliced tomatoes, pickles (avoid if on a low-sodium diet), beet salad, or carrot-raisin salad.

Worst Choices

Obviously, there are many unhealthy choices lurking in the columns of the deli menu. Those to avoid are the high-fat meats: regular corned beef and hot pastrami, beef bologna, salami, knockwurst, hot dogs, liverwurst, and tongue. Also steer away from combination sandwiches that have upwards of six ounces of meat unless you are planning on sharing. Reuben sandwiches are grilled, contain corned beef, cheese, and Russian dressing, are topped with either coleslaw or, more authentically, sauerkraut—a fat and sodium nightmare!

Other common delicatessen listings to veer away from are the smoked fishes—lox, whitefish salad, and smoked sable fish. Avoid chopped liver, creamy coleslaw, potato salad, and large portions of cream cheese, chive cheese, and lox or veggie cream cheese spread.

SUBMARINE SHOPS

Depending on what part of the country you grew up in, those long sandwich rolls filled with all sorts of high-fat meats—salami, bologna, mortadella—and topped with cheeses—provolone and mozzarella—might be known as subs, hoagies, heros, or grinders. Whatever the name, these sandwiches are familiar to the American diner. Philadelphia puts itself on the map with its well known Philadelphia cheese steaks, which are served in submarine rolls. Philadelphia cheese steaks are no longer just served in the City of Brotherly Love; they've spread their fame across the country. Unfortunately, the famous cheese-steak sandwiches are not among the healthiest of food choices.

Subs (the term I'm most familiar with) are frequently served in small family-run restaurants, where pizza and salads are also on the menu. Also, many large chains exist across the country whose main business is serving up those long submarine sandwiches. A big chain in the New England area called D'Angelo's simply serves subs, pocket sandwiches, and a variety of salads. Their menu even has a "delicious and lowest in calories" section.

It's no longer true that you'll only find Italian meats and cheeses packed into the thick submarine roll. Today, there are many different fillings used such as seafood or tuna salad, turkey, roast beef, or hot ham. Also in many sub shops you have a choice between the big sub roll or Syrian pocket (pita) bread. And there are size choices: small, medium, or large. The broader selection means that sub shops can be an acceptable pick for a lunch spot.

However, it's still important to choose carefully. Fat, saturated fat, cholesterol, and sodium are your enemies—mainly contributed by the stuff between the bread. Once again, the bread and toppings, lettuce, tomato, onions, pickles, and hot peppers are the healthiest part of a sub. It might come as a surprise, but a roast beef sub is a far better choice than a tuna-fish sub. According to USDA nutrient analysis, a roast beef sub has around 400 calories, with 30 percent from fat, and about 850 milligrams of sodium. In comparison, a tunafish salad sub has almost 600 calories, with 43 percent from fat. It also has a whopping 1,300 milligrams of sodium. The cholesterol is a bit lower for the tuna sub, but both are under 75 milligrams. So even though we see the healthy word "fish" in tuna-fish salad, it's laden with fat before it reaches your plate.

Best Choices

Let's consider the best choices in a sub shop. If you've got some calories to spare, go ahead and have the small-size sub roll. This will help fill you up and give you a good dose of carbos. If your calorie budget is tighter, have a Syrian pita pocket. They usually use about two-thirds of the pocket, which puts the sandwich in the range of 150 calories, probably half of what's in the small sub roll. The best meats to order are turkey, smoked turkey, roast beef, ham, and hot ham (this is a great spicy choice). Use a limited amount of cheese, and only if you're not closely monitoring saturated fat and cholesterol intake.

Make sure to load up on fresh veggies. I'll usually ask that the preparer go light on the meats, hold the oil or mayonnaise, and load on the shredded lettuce, sliced tomatoes, onions, pickles, and hot peppers. The pickles and hot peppers will definitely add some sodium, but if that's not a big concern, have them piled on—they add great spicy flavor.

There are several salads to choose from as an alternative to the sub sandwich. These are commonly served with Italian bread or half a Syrian pocket. The usuals are tossed garden, chef salad, antipasto, Greek salad, and tossed salad offered with a scoop of tuna, chicken, or seafood. On some menus you'll find tossed or Greek salad served in a pita pocket. The tossed, chef (with some substitutes for lower-fat items if necessary), Greek, and tuna, chicken, or seafood salads, if you've got a few extra calories to spare, are fine choices. An antipasto, with all its high-fat and sodium ingredients, is best avoided. Remember, the biggest nutrition pitfall with salads is the type and amount of dressing used. Generally speaking, use less and use the lower or no-calorie varieties (vinegar is always available). For more tips on the use of salad dressings, review Chapter 15 on salad bars.

OK Choices

If you've got a few more calories and a bit more fat to work with, there are a few OK choices in sub shops.

Steak and onions, mushrooms, and/or peppers in a sub roll or pocket sandwich are a few. Stay away from steak and cheese; that's just adding insult to injury. The tuna salad and other usual salads—seafood, shrimp, or chicken—are OK in a sub or on a garden salad, but the fat content is certainly higher than the unadulterated lower-fat meats that have no extra fat added in the form of mayonnaise.

Worst Choices

There are, of course, several items to avoid. Among this group are bologna, hard or Genoa salami, mortadella (Italian cold cut), cheeses, sausage (which is often combined with sauteed vegetables), steak and cheese, eggplant (always fried and usually combined with cheeses), chicken cutlet, and chicken or veal parmigiana. The last three listings start off sounding healthy, but they are frequently deep-fried, and parmigiana means topped with cheese.

FOOD COURTS & MALL EATERIES

To make sure we Americans are always secure knowing that there is food nearby, the food courts have been a new addition to malls in many cities. The newer large malls are being built with eatery sections, and older malls may be renovated to offer various bites to eat.

The size of these food courts and the diversity of restaurants varies. The food court in the newly renovated Union Station, located in Washington, DC, about a block from our nation's capitol building, offers members of the U.S. Congress and their staffs (as well as other citizens) almost any type of ethnic cuisine along with good old American fare. Actually, renovated train stations are found in several other cities. They also contain a broad array of fast foods and casual dining—St. Louis and Indianapolis are two examples. Smaller eatery sections are found in many shopping malls around the country.

Food courts offer a few advantages. Food is served quickly: you simply stand in line, order, and take it to a table. Another advantage is that if you are dining with a group, everyone has an opportunity to choose their favorite lunch spots, then regroup and have lunch together.

One of the biggest drawbacks to the food courts, as one of my weight-control clients brought to mind, is that there are tremendous visual and taste stimuli and way too many choices. For those who have a difficult time making decisions and avoiding the "danger" foods, mall eateries can be overwhelming. These folks might do best by detouring food courts. If you choose a mall eatery due to convenience, or group decision, the best advice is to have a firm plan in mind prior to arriving.

The common restaurant choices in mall eateries are the standard American fare–hamburgers and fries, fried chicken, hot dogs, sub sandwiches, salad bars, and stuffed potatoes. There's also plenty of popular ethnic fare–Italian spaghetti and pizza, Mexican tacos and burritos, Chinese eggrolls, fried rice, and chop suey, and Middle Eastern food with gyros, falafel, and tabooli. In the larger eateries you might find a sushi bar, fruit and frozen yogurt stands, bakeries, and confections.

After discovering Union Station in Washington, I looked over the situation in my usual quest for a relatively nutritious spot to have lunch and happened upon Pikapita, billed as naturally fresh fast food. Pikapita lived up to its claim; they had some delightful low-fat, healthy choices such as roasted chicken or beef rolled in a pita with lettuce and fattoush, a salad served with light lemon-garlic dressing and pita chips. This convinced me that among the nutritional disasters at food courts are other, healthier choices.

Good, OK, and Worst Choices

When contemplating about which direction is best to take when you enter a food court, keep the following thoughts in mind. Look for a place serving fresh, unadulterated foods: fruit cups with or without frozen yogurt, salad bars, sub sandwiches, Greek salad at the Middle Eastern spot, or stuffed baked potatoes. Avoid the fried foods: fried chicken, French fries, deep-fried vegetables, fried fish, and high-fat choices that include lots of red meats and cheeses. For more details on good choices at food courts, refer to the specific ethnic cuisine. For instance, if Chinese food is your choice of the day, consult Chapter 5, "Healthier Eating Out: Chinese Style," for some smart selections.

WORK-SITE CAFETERIAS

Many people find themselves at lunch, perhaps even breakfast or dinner, depending on which shift they work, in the employee cafeteria day after day. In my travels through many different work sites I've seen the gamut, from very limited choices of soups, sandwiches, and pre-packaged tossed salad (if you're lucky) to employee cafeterias with an elaborate array of choices—hot items, a wide selection of cold as well as grilled sandwiches, a well-stocked salad bar, yogurts, plenty of fresh fruit, and tempting desserts.

The benefit of frequenting the employee cafeteria for lunch is that it's a known entity—there are few surprises. You know what the offerings will be prior to your arrival. Thus, you can have a game plan before entering.

Another benefit of being a somewhat captive audience is that you can make some special requests for foods you'd like to see among the cafeteria's healthier choices. Employers today are, hopefully, concerned about their employees' health, if for no other reason than the fact that providing health insurance benefits to employees is costly. Most companies today have some interest in keeping you healthy.

For starters, discuss your wants and desires with the cafeteria manager. Perhaps you should take several of your coworkers along so the manager realizes there's a consensus. Be specific and realistic about the healthier foods you'd like available. Maybe it's lower-fat yogurt or a non-fat yogurt machine, lower-calorie salad dressings on the salad bar, balsamic vinegar, or Syrian pita pockets as a bread choice at the sandwich bar. These are all easy requests to meet. If talking to the cafeteria manager doesn't work, try the employer health nurse or medical department. The people who assist in keeping you healthy might be willing to help.

Another benefit of eating lunch in the work-site cafeteria is that it's perfectly acceptable to bring part or all of your lunch. In the long run this technique keeps more change in your pockets. So use this tactic by bringing some healthier items from home if they are not available in the cafeteria.

Perhaps you have a favorite low-calorie salad dressing, and the cafeteria doesn't stock it. Keep your bottle at work, and just take it to the cafeteria when you're having a salad. Flip-top individual servings of tunafish are available now and would be great to bring and toss on top of the salad you purchase from the cafeteria. Most likely the cafeteria will only have tuna made into tuna salad, with lots of mayonnaise. It's easy to grab a piece of fruit from home, which may help complete your meal, and avoid going for the sweet treats that usually aren't worth the calories. Maybe you'll bring a sandwich from home and complement it with the cooked vegetable offering of the day.

Once again, you need to pick and choose wisely in the employee cafeteria. There will be good, OK, and poor choices at most work-site cafeterias, large or small. Apply the rules of thumb that have been suggested under Sandwich Shops, Delicatessens, and Submarine Shops. Many of these same food selections will be available at most cafeterias. If you often use the salad bar, consult Chapter 15 on "Healthier Eating Out: Salad Bar Style."

Typical Menu: Luncheon Style

Soups   **New England clam chowder**
              (creamy chowder filled with
              minced clams and potatoes)
              ✓**Chili** (thick spicy chili chock full
              of beef and beans)
              ✓**Vegetable soup** (light, brothy
              soup filled with fresh vegetables)

Salads* ✓**House salad** (lettuce topped with
              peppers, mushrooms, cucumbers,
              and tomatoes)
              ✓**Spinach salad** (spinach leaves
              topped with sliced mushrooms, ba-
              con bits, sliced egg, and bean
              sprouts)
              ✓**Greek salad** (bed of lettuce
              topped with crumbled feta cheese,
              red onions, and Greek olives)
              ✓**Chef salad** (bed of greens topped
              with ham, turkey, Swiss cheese,
              tomatoes, and cucumbers)
              **Tuna, chicken, or seafood
              salad** (bed of greens with tomato,
              green peppers, and bean sprouts
              topped with a scoop of tuna,
              chicken, or seafood salad)
              ✓**Roasted chicken salad** (roasted
              chicken sliced on bed of romaine
              lettuce, sliced tomato, and
              cucumber)

              *Salad served with choice of
              dressing: blue cheese, Thousand
              Island, Italian, French, ranch,
              ✓lemon-garlic, or ✓low-calorie
              Italian.

✓*Preferred Choice*

Luncheon Style

Cold Sandwiches*	✓Smoked turkey ✓Turkey breast ✓Roast beef Egg salad Chicken salad Tuna salad Seafood salad Hot pastrami ✓Corned beef ✓Ham and cheese ✓Turkey and cheese Club sandwich (choice of turkey or roast beef)
Hot Sandwiches*	Reuben (corned beef grilled with cheese and sauerkraut, topped with Thousand Island dressing) ✓Hamburgers (plain or topped with choice or combination of cheese, bacon, or chili) Grilled cheese (with tomatoes and/or bacon) ✓Grilled chicken breast ✓Bacon, lettuce, and tomato Grilled hot dog Tuna melt (scoop of tuna salad with melted mozzarella cheese) ✓Veggie cheese melt (sauteed mushrooms, peppers, and onions topped with melted Swiss cheese) *All sandwiches can be made on a choice of: ✓submarine roll, white, ✓whole-wheat, or ✓pumpernickel bread, ✓kaiser roll, croissant, or ✓Syrian pocket. All sandwiches can be made with lettuce, tomatoes, and/or onions and are served with pickles.
Combinations	✓Soup and salad (cup of any soup served with House or Spinach salad) ✓Soup and half-sandwich (cup of any soup served with choice of cold sandwich)

✓**Salad and half-sandwich** (House Salad served with choice of cold sandwich)

Side **French fries**
Orders **Onion rings**
✓**Tabooli salad**
✓**Coleslaw**
Potato salad
Macaroni salad
✓**Plain yogurt**
Potato chips
✓**Popcorn**
Corn chips
✓**Pretzels**

Desserts **Chocolate-chip cookies**
Chocolate cake
Apple pie
✓**Fresh fruit cup**
✓**Assorted fresh fruits**

Now that you've seen what may be available on lunch menus, look over the following five "Model Meals" for suggestions on how to order to achieve specific nutritional goals. Models are numbered one to five for quick reference, and each is followed by an "Estimated Nutrient Evaluation" that analyzes the content of that meal.

May I Take Your Order*

Healthy	30% Calories as fat
Daily	20% Calories as protein
Eating	50% Calories as carbohydrate
Goals	300 mg/day Cholesterol
	3000 mg/day Sodium

❶
Low Calorie/
Low Fat
Model Meal

(From typical Food Court/Mall Eatery menu)

Roasted chicken salad (dressing on the side)
Quantity: 3 oz meat; 2 cups salad
Exchanges: 3 meat (lean); 2 vegetables
Dressing: (on the side)
Quantity: 2 tbsp
Exchanges: 1 fat
Tabooli salad with lemon-herb dressing
Quantity: ½ cup
Exchanges: 1 fat; 1 starch
Apple (brought from home)
Quantity: 1 small
Exchanges: 1 fruit
Mineral water
Quantity: 10 oz
Exchanges: free

Estimated
Nutrient
Evaluation

425 calories
21% calories as fat
33% calories as protein
46% calories as carbohydrate
73 mg cholesterol
862 mg sodium

❷
Low Calorie/ Low Cholesterol Model Meal

(From typical Delicatessen menu)

Smoked turkey sandwich with lettuce, tomato, onion, and mustard (eat half; share half)
Quantity: 3 oz meat, 2 slices bread
Pumpernickel bread for above
Quantity: 2 slices
Pickle (avoid if on low-sodium diet)
Quantity: ½
Coleslaw
Quantity: ¾ cup
Low-calorie carbonated beverage
Quantity: 12 oz

Estimated Nutrient Evaluation

464 calories
28% calories as fat
26% calories as protein
46% calories as carbohydrate
92 mg cholesterol
1712 mg sodium (998 without pickle)

❸
Higher Calorie/Low Fat Model Meal

(From typical Submarine Shop menu)

Roast beef sub with lettuce, tomato, onion, pickle, and hot peppers (hold the oil)
Quantity: 1 small sub with 2 cups toppings
Exchanges: 4 meat (lean); 2 vegetable; 2 starches
Popcorn
Quantity: ¾ oz
Exchanges: 1 fat; 1 starch
Iced tea
Exchanges: free

Estimated Nutrient Evaluation	588 calories
	28% calories as fat
	24% calories as protein
	48% calories as carbohydrate
	76 mg cholesterol
	1405 mg sodium (reduce by avoiding pickles and hot peppers)

---

❹
Higher Calorie/Low Cholesterol Model Meal

(From typical Sandwich Shop menu)

Vegetable soup
Quantity: 1 cup
Grilled chicken breast sandwich with lettuce, tomato, and mustard
Quantity: 3 oz meat
Syrian pocket for above
Quantity: ⅔ whole pocket
Fresh fruit cup
Quantity: ¾ cup
Milk, low-fat (skim preferable)
Quantity: 1 cup

Estimated Nutrient Evaluation	589 calories
	16% calories as fat
	31% calories as protein
	53% calories as carbohydrate
	73 mg cholesterol
	1437 mg sodium (800 accounted for by soup)

---

❺
Low Sodium Model Meal

(From typical Work-Site Cafeteria menu)

Salad bar: lettuce, tomato, red onion, alfalfa sprouts
Quantity: 2–3 cups
Pickled beets
Quantity: ¼ cup
Chick peas
Quantity: ¼ cup

Tuna salad
Quantity: ½ cup
Low-calorie Italian dressing
Quantity: 2 tbsp
Pear
Quantity: 1 small
Milk, skim
Quantity: 1 cup

Estimated
Nutrient
Evaluation

   593 calories
22% calories as fat
30% calories as protein
48% calories as carbohydrate
  39 mg cholesterol
857 mg sodium (using vinegar instead of salad dressing would reduce to 600 mg)

*Note: These model meals were developed to be slightly lower in calories and other major nutrients than model meals in other chapters because lunch is often a lower-calorie meal than dinner.

17

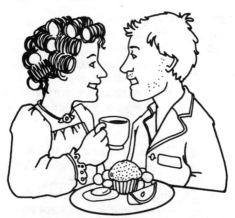

Healthier eating out

Breakfast and Brunch

L ate for work, on vacation, on a business trip, it's Sunday morning, driving along the highway, or celebrating with a champagne brunch—just a few reasons why breakfast or brunch is eaten away from home. The National Restaurant Association's most recent figures indicate that approximately 18 percent of consumers eat breakfast out at least once a week, even though breakfast is the meal least frequently eaten out. However, in our fast-paced world, it's hard to believe that the number of people consuming breakfast out is not on the rise. Granted, your definition of breakfast might be grabbing a bite at the corner muffin shop, stopping by the convenience store, or driving through a fast food spot on the way to work, school, or wherever.

Another reason breakfast is the meal least frequently eaten out is because it's the most frequently skipped meal. Everyone has heard the gospel about breakfast from dietitians and health care professionals: "Breakfast is the most important meal of the day," "it gives you a good start on the day," "it provides energy to complete your morning activities." Think about the word "BREAK FAST"; it literally means to "break the fast," that is, the overnight fast.

Unfortunately, the vicious cycle that many people, especially those who struggle with excess pounds, get into is as follows: the alarm clock goes off, the snooze alarm is hit (once, if not several times), now you're late, you make the mad dash to be on time, and, as usual, there's no time for breakfast. As the day goes on, maybe you grab lunch. When you get home, you are starving, and often one large meal is consumed from the time the door is unlocked until your head hits the pillow. The nighttime overeating is rationalized by the minimal calories consumed during the day. Unfortunately, you have just consumed the bulk of your calories when your body least needs them and when your metabolic rate is slowing down.

Newer health and weight control information is more solidly touting the benefits of breakfast than ever before. Eating breakfast seems to press the button to get your metabolism in gear. If you don't eat, your metabolism doesn't get the jump-start it needs. So as the morning rolls on and you don't feed your body, you send the message that you are fasting. Your metabolic rate responds by remaining sluggish. Evidence indicates that people who eat breakfast are more likely to be at a desired body weight.

We'd all be better off if more calories were consumed in the morning or whenever the body is doing the most work. Caloric intake should be tapered off when the body starts slowing down for the resting and relaxing part of the day. Due to many factors, that is difficult for many of us.

A wise health and waist-watcher goal is to eat something for breakfast no matter what healthy foods you choose. A slice of last night's pizza, eaten cold, is better than a mid-morning bag of chips and can of regular soda. It doesn't have to be a traditional, hearty breakfast to be healthy. In fact, you're better off avoiding some traditional American breakfast foods as we'll see.

Nutritional trouble spots at breakfast time

Eggs, bacon strips, sausage patties, omelettes, muffins, toast with butter, bagels and cream cheese, pancakes and waffles topped with whipped butter and syrup are all foods that come to mind when you hear the words "breakfast" or "brunch." As this list of foods is reviewed, you'll see that many don't fit today's prescription for healthy foods. Several start out moderately healthy—toast, bagels, muffins, and pancakes and waffles—but usually end up eaten slathered with various fats. Calories and cholesterol are boosted significantly.

The traditional American breakfast of eggs, bacon or sausage, pancakes, etc., traces back to the days when the majority of Americans were farming. By the time people ate breakfast, they had practically done a day's work. People working the land did, and continue to burn significantly more calories than those of us involved in the high-tech world. Interestingly though, the traditional, diehard eggs, bacon, etc., continue to appear most frequently on breakfast and brunch menus.

Take a moment to consider the nutrition breakdown of the following traditional breakfast:

4 oz orange juice
2 eggs, scrambled
2 slices of bacon
2 slices of toast; 2 teaspoons of butter
½ cup of home fries
1 oz light cream for coffee

This breakfast has approximately 730 calories, with 53 percent of them coming from fat, and almost 280 milligrams of cholesterol. About enough cholesterol to meet the entire day's goal.

This example is not even the worst of American breakfast regulars. Consider one of Denny's grand-slam breakfast offerings: 2 large pancakes (served with butter and maple syrup), 2 eggs, 2 strips of bacon, and 2 sausage links. Estimate the calorie, fat, and cholesterol content of that meal!

Pancakes, waffles, and French toast are additional American breakfast and brunch favorites. They start off relatively healthy but typically have butter or margarine and syrup poured on top. Also, they're commonly served with bacon, sausage, ham, or Canadian bacon—all adding more protein, fat, and calories. Obviously, you can request that the breakfast meats be omitted.

Brunches are supposed to be a combination of breakfast and lunch, but based on the nutritional content of most brunches, they should do the trick for dinner as well! This is especially true for the all-you-can-eat brunches. Eggs Benedict, consisting of 2 eggs on English muffins, Canadian bacon, and all topped with hollandaise sauce, is a favorite. Omelettes are another brunch favorite. Often there's a chef making omelettes to order with your choice of ingredients.

Most restaurants tout that their omelettes are made with three farm-fresh eggs. Using the newest USDA figures for eggs, there's 213 milligrams of cholesterol in each, which puts you at 639 milligrams just for the eggs. Then most omelettes add other protein, cholesterol and fat-containing ingredients—cheese, ham, bacon, or sauteed vegetables. An omelette can be upward of 400–500 calories before you add the hash browns, toast and butter, or bagel and cream cheese.

Fast food breakfasts have become very popular due in large part to our fast-paced society. As you might imagine, they're also trouble spots for calories and fat. The ever-popular Egg McMuffin, served by McDonald's, is really one of the better offerings. It's about 300 calories, and 35 percent of the calories are from fat. Due to the egg, it provides the better part of your daily cholesterol allotment. On the worst choice list, Jack-in-the-Box offers its Sausage Crescent Sandwich, which has 580 calories, 66 percent from fat. It also provides slightly over 1,000 milligrams of sodium. Each fast food spot has its better and worst choices. A table is provided at the end of this chapter, containing "Nutrition Information on Selected Fast Food Breakfast Choices."

Even though the foods that first come to mind when breakfast is mentioned don't win any nutritional gold medals, there are many foods frequently appearing on restaurant menus that assist you in eating a healthier breakfast. Cereals, hot or cold; high-fiber toast or muffins; and yogurt and fresh fruit are just a few.

The wide range of breakfast and brunch spots

Possibly among the most popular breakfast spots in today's get-the-job-done-quickly world are the muffin, doughnut, and bagel shops. Sometimes they're all in one. People flock in by the dozens and order a muffin, doughnut, or bagel with whatever spread. A beverage, commonly coffee but maybe tea or juice, is also an essential part of the order. Then it's off to the place of employment to gulp down breakfast while initiating the daily tasks.

As fast food grows in popularity, so do fast food breakfasts. Most of the chains have several breakfast offerings, ranging from a sandwich of sorts to eggs, pancakes, and French toast. In 1976 McDonald's was first on the fast food breakfast scene with its Egg McMuffin. As usual, they found themselves the leader in a new marketplace for the fast food industry. A *Time* magazine article of August 26, 1985, notes that breakfast is the "newest fast food battleground." As of 1985, breakfast represented 19.5 percent of total sales for McDonald's. The article goes on to state that "fast food executives see breakfast as a lucrative area for expansion. Mornings are a time when Americans are usually in a rush."

Hotels, both in big cities and on America's highways, usually offer a breakfast menu. On a business trip, at a convention, doing some early morning driving, or just enjoying a relaxing vacation, you might find yourself at a hotel or motel restaurant. Typically, you'll find menu listings of cereal, eggs, pancakes, French toast, Danish, and others. Sometimes, you'll see a buffet offered at the large hotels. This requires less labor, and it enables them to feed many people in a quick fashion. Recently, I was at a convention in Detroit, and the Westin offered a hot or cold buffet. The cold buffet offered some great, healthy choices: yogurt, fresh fruit, small muffins, toast, and a selection of cold cereals.

It's common to see elaborate brunch buffets served in large downtown hotels on weekends. The food choices can range from a chef making omelettes to a chef slicing roast beef to a wide selection of breads from toast and bagels to croissants and sweet rolls. In addition, many weekend brunches offer champagne, mimosas, and Bloody Marys—the traditional morning alcoholic beverages. They usually have a set price, and it's "all you can eat." Unfortunately, you do eat all you can and come out with that post-Thanksgiving dinner feeling—like a stuffed turkey.

Many people also enjoy breakfast at truck stops along the highway or in good-old-times coffee shops along the streets of small and large towns. The offerings in these spots are similar to those in hotel restaurants. The grill is usually in a predominant spot, and you see eggs being scrambled or fried, bacon or sausage grilling, and the toast popping up and being brushed with melted butter. Cold and hot cereals are among the selections.

Delicatessens are also popular breakfast spots. During the work week, it's common to stop in for a bagel topped with some cream cheese mixture—maybe veggie, chive, or lox spread. Whereas on the weekend it's more usual to see people enjoying a scramble of lox, eggs, and onions, which I've been told is more familiarly referred to as a LEO. A bagel with white fish salad, a smoked fish plate, or blintzes served with sour cream are also common orders. Unfortunately, most of these choices result in breakfasts or brunches that derive 50 percent or more of their calories from fat.

Many cities and towns also have one, two, or more pancake or waffle houses. Probably the most well known across America is the International House of Pancakes, or IHOP, as it is abbreviated. Waffle House is another well-known breakfast chain. These spots offer a wide range of pancakes, waffles, and French toast with various toppings and accompaniments of bacon, sausage, or ham. Eggs, toast, etc., are frequently part of the menu listings.

No matter what restaurant you chose or where you happen to be at breakfast time, there are always healthy choices, be it in a coffee shop, muffin stop, or Jewish deli. You might need to begin by redefining breakfast and then trying some of the healthier, lower-fat, and lower-cholesterol options.

Breakfast and Brunch

What to consider before ordering

We tend to think of breakfast as the lowest calorie and lightest meal of the day—just picking up a muffin or bagel or buzzing by the nearest fast food spot for a simple egg, cheese, and ham sandwich. In reality the story is quite different. As you've read, the food choices might be small in volume, but they pack quite a bit of fat and calories. If you're watching your weight, as most of us are, you might be trying to maintain a daily calorie intake in the range of 1,200 to 1,800 calories. If you use in excess of 600 calories for breakfast, that makes it difficult to stay within the daily goals.

Granted, it would be great if you ate more at breakfast and tapered off the rest of the day. However, that's not the pattern most Americans follow. For many, simply eating something for breakfast is a move in the direction of health and weight control. Taking a realistic approach, try shooting for the goal of consuming 20–30 percent of your calories at breakfast. Strive to keep the carbohydrates up and the protein and fat down. If you load up on protein in the A.M. from two eggs or a cheese omelette, you'll have a rough time keeping within your protein allotment for the day. That's not even mentioning the excess fat and cholesterol. Try to keep the fat to 20–25 percent of total calorie intake. That means going for cereals, fruits, yogurt, and breads with jellies and jams. All these choices leave out most of the fat.

As for those weekend "all-you-can-eat" brunches, the best advice is to avoid them. Steer your dining companions in the direction of a restaurant with a menu. That way you can order healthy items without being surrounded with foods that are crying to be eaten and feeling guilty that you are wasting money.

If your arm is twisted or you believe in self-torture and you're at an all-you-can-eat spread, follow a few rules of thumb. First, survey the situation—check out what foods are available. Plan what you will choose and in what quantity. Try a bowl of fresh fruit or salad—that will take the edge off your appetite. Then only allow yourself one trip to the buffet. If you want to taste numerous items, take small quantities. Lastly, drink plenty of fluids, enjoy the relaxing environment, and get some extra exercise beforehand or after you've digested the brunch.

Managing the menu

The start to breakfast is often the automatic glass of orange juice. Few people are aware that even a six-ounce glass of almost any juice provides at least 80 calories. Don't get me wrong, those are healthy calories, but you'd be better off *eating* fruit rather than slurping it quickly. Try ordering a half-grapefruit, slice of melon, or fresh fruit instead of the usual glass of juice. Fruit will provide more fiber, more volume, and simply take you longer to eat. Fruit can also be used on cereal or on pancakes, French toast, or waffles in place of the high-calorie butter and syrup.

Cold cereals are almost always available at breakfast restaurants. Often you've got several to choose from—Cornflakes, Puffed Wheat, Shredded Wheat, Rice Krispies, Raisin Bran, and Bran Flakes are among the regulars. It's best to use the whole-grain cereals; they provide more fiber. Almost all cold cereals, sugar coated or not, contain sugar or a form of sugar among the top four ingredients. People who have diabetes are told they can choose from any of the non-sugar-coated cereals. However, several have no sugar at all added, such as Shredded Wheat, Puffed Wheat, and Puffed Rice. Surprisingly, cold cereals have a chunk of sodium, on average about 250 milligrams.

Hot cereals are usually among the menu listings. Either oatmeal or cream of wheat are often available. Again, it's great to use the oat-based cereals to increase soluble fiber intake. Maybe we will soon see oat bran cereals appearing on menus. Hot cereals as well as cold cereals offer mainly carbohydrates and no fat (unless it is added).

Obviously, you're best off topping your cereal with low-fat or, better yet, skim milk. Low fat is about the best you can do in most restaurants. Avoid the whole milk and cream. Top cold or hot cereal with bananas or other fresh fruit.

Pancakes, French toast, and waffles are basically made from the same ingredients: flour, water, egg, a bit of sugar, and a leavening agent. Before the whipped butter and syrup are loaded on, they're really not nutritional disasters. Unfortunately, the portions are often way more than you need. To solve that problem, share an order or order a "short stack" of pancakes. If you ask the waitperson to hold the butter and you use only a bit of syrup, or top with fresh fruit, jam, jelly, or sugar substitute and cinnamon (especially good on French toast), their healthiness dramatically improves.

Guidelines of the American Heart Association and other health organizations advise no more than 3–5 egg yolks per week. The largest problem with eggs is their cholesterol content, at 213 milligrams per egg. It all comes from the yolk. However, eggs are moderate in their saturated fat content. The biggest problem with ordering eggs in restaurants is that they usually come in duplicate or triplicate. It's best to avoid the omelettes unless you're sharing a veggie one. If you're due for an egg, try ordering just one. Poaching requires no fat, whereas fat is used to scramble or fry an egg.

There are often numerous choices from the bread and bakery category—some smart and others better left on the baker's shelf. Let's start with the increasingly popular muffin. Unfortunately, muffins have received quite a bit of hype due to the emphasis on increasing fiber intake. A recent article in the May, 1989, issue of the *Tufts Diet and Nutrition Newsletter* entitled "Making Sense Out of Muffin Mania" provides some enlightening information about the current muffin craze. In relation to fiber, they state ". . . most bran muffins . . . have about as much fiber as you would get in a half-cup to a cup of many branflake cereals. The cereals, unlike the muffins, have little if any fat, however."

Tufts' analysis of several national store-bought brands and some available from doughnut shops, such as Dunkin' Donuts, reveals that on average the 3–3½-ounce (on the large side) muffin contains in the range of 250–450 calories, about 30–35 percent of which come from fat. Surprisingly, the "healthier, high-fiber muffins" are not what they're cracked up to be. However, if you have a moderate-size bran or oat bran muffin without any added fats, then add a piece of fruit, that's a quick and reasonably healthy choice. Note the nutrient analysis for the low calorie/low cholesterol breakfast under "May I Take Your Order."

It's best to avoid the high-fat croissants, biscuits, Danish, doughnuts (especially deep-fried as opposed to cake type), and coffeecakes. Healthy breakfast breads, which contain ostensibly no fat, are toast, bagels, and English muffins. If you can choose wholegrain varieties, all the better.

The next step is to be careful about what you load on top. Request that any bread be served dry. Keep margarine, butter, cream cheese, and other fats to a minimum. Use the jams and jellies instead. For people with diabetes who should avoid jams and jellies, it might be wise to carry some of the prepackaged no-sugar-added jellies, that is, until restaurants start serving the all-fruit spreads that are widely available in the supermarket.

The breakfast accompaniments can often add to the fat content. Think about the bacon, sausage, ham, or Canadian bacon that is served alongside eggs, pancakes, and French toast. They all add fat, sodium, and significant calories. The best of the choices, unless you are carefully monitoring sodium consumption, are ham and Canadian bacon because they are leaner. But it's best to avoid them all.

Breakfast potatoes, whether they are called hash browns or home fries, are another example of taking a great food—potatoes—and adding fat and sodium in the cooking process. The fast food varieties of breakfast potatoes derive at least 55 percent of their calories from fat. (Observe the fast food table at the end of the chapter.) Ask how the potatoes are prepared. If they are homemade, they might be lighter in fat content than the pre-formed frozen and deep-fried potatoes.

Side orders appearing more frequently are yogurt and cottage cheese. Both can be healthy additions to any breakfast. Use these to top off fruit or breakfast breads. You might do best ordering à la carte, though it's not always economical. Try fresh fruit, yogurt, or cottage cheese and whole-wheat toast or a bagel. Or share an order of pancakes, French toast, or waffles and order yogurt and fresh fruit à la carte as a topping.

Typical Menu: Breakfast and Brunch

Fruits and Juices	✓**Juices,** small or large (orange, grapefruit, apple, cranberry, tomato) ✓**Grapefruit half** ✓**Fresh fruit cup** ✓**Sliced melon**
Cereals*	✓**Cold cereal** (Cornflakes, Special K, Raisin Bran, Bran Flakes) **Granola** (a natural, oat-based cereal filled with nuts and grains) ✓**Hot cereal** (Oatmeal, Cream of Wheat, Cream of Rice, Wheatena) *Served with cream, whole milk, or low-fat milk on the side. All cereals also available with fresh fruit.
Pancakes, French Toast, Waffles	✓**Buttermilk pancakes,** stack of 3 large* ✓**Silver dollar pancakes** (10–12 small buttermilk pancakes)* ✓**Blueberry pancakes** (3 large buttermilk pancakes filled with blueberries, topped with whipped butter, and served with blueberry syrup) **French toast** (4 halves of extra-thick bread, dipped in egg batter, and grilled)* ✓**Belgian waffle*** **Belgian waffle with strawberries** (thick Belgian waffle topped with strawberry sauce and whipped cream) *Served with whipped butter on top and syrup on the side. All available with choice of bacon, sausage links, or sausage patties.

✓*Preferred Choice*

Eggs*   ✓**One egg** (fried, scrambled, or poached)
Two eggs (fried, scrambled, or poached)
Eggs Benedict (two English muffin halves, each topped with Canadian bacon, poached egg, and hollandaise sauce)
Eggs Grecian (2 eggs baked with spinach, onions, and crumbled feta cheese, served topped with cream sauce)
Steak and eggs (2 eggs prepared to order and served with 8-oz sirloin strip)

*All egg dishes served with choice of bacon, sausage links, or ham plus home fries and 2 slices of buttered toast.

Omelettes*   **Western** with sauteed onions and green peppers; covered with Cheddar cheese and diced ham)
Florentine (filled with spinach, onions, and feta cheese; topped with creamy mushroom sauce)
Three-cheese omelette (combination of Cheddar, Swiss, and Muenster)
✓**Veggie** (filled with sauteed onions, green and red peppers, and mushrooms; topped with Swiss cheese)

*All omelettes made with 3 eggs and served with choice of bacon, sausage patties, or Canadian bacon plus hash browns and 2 slices of buttered toast.

Breads/ **Bakery**	**Croissant** ✓**Muffin** (choice of blueberry, raisin bran, or oat bran) ✓**Bagel** (choice of plain, onion, or raisin; served with cream cheese) **Danish pastry** (choice of apple or cheese) **Doughnut** (honey-dipped or cinnamon) ✓**Biscuit** ✓**Toast** (choice of white, whole-wheat, rye, or pumpernickel) ✓**English muffin**
Side **Orders**	**Bacon** **Sausage,** links or patties ✓**Ham** ✓**Canadian bacon** ✓**Home fries** **Hash browns** **Cream cheese** ✓**Cottage cheese** ✓**Fruited yogurt** ✓**Plain yogurt**

Now that you've seen what may be available on the breakfast or brunch menu, look over the following five "Model Meals" for suggestions on how to order to achieve specific nutritional goals. Models are numbered one to five for quick reference, and each is followed by an "Estimated Nutrient Evaluation" that analyzes the content of that meal.

*May I Take Your Order**

Healthy Daily Eating Goals	30% Calories as fat 20% Calories as protein 50% Calories as carbohydrate 300 mg Cholesterol 3000 mg Sodium

❶
Low Calorie/
Low Fat
Model Meal

(From typical Coffee Shop menu)

Banana, sliced
Quantity: ½
Exchanges: 1 fruit
Cold or Hot cereal (high-fiber,
    bran, oatmeal, or oat bran)
Quantity: 1 box or 1 cup
Exchanges: 1½ starch
Milk, low-fat (skim preferable)
Quantity: 1 cup
Exchanges: 1 milk

Estimated
Nutrient
Evaluation

272 calories
13% calories as fat
16% calories as protein
71% calories as carbohydrate
  18 mg cholesterol
342 mg sodium

❷
Low Calorie/
Low
Cholesterol
Model Meal

(From typical Doughnut Shop menu)

Muffin, bran, oat bran, or raisin
  bran
Quantity: 1 small
Fresh fruit (from home)
Quantity: 1 small serving

Estimated Nutrient Evaluation	393 calories
	30% calories as fat
	9% calories as protein
	61% calories as carbohydrate
	0–20 mg cholesterol (depending on fat used in muffin)
	550 mg sodium

---

❸

Higher Calorie/Low Fat Model Meal

(From typical Delicatessen menu)

Orange juice
Quantity: 6 oz
Exchanges: 1½ fruit
Egg, poached
Quantity: 1
Exchanges: 1 meat (med.)
Bagel (cream cheese on the side)
Quantity: 1 small
Exchanges: 2 starch
Veggie cream cheese for above
Quantity: 1 tbsp
Exchanges: 1 fat
Home fries
Quantity: ½ cup
Exchanges: 1 fat; 1 starch

Estimated Nutrient Evaluation	541 calories
	37% calories as fat
	12% calories as protein
	51% calories as carbohydrate
	228 mg cholesterol
	560 mg sodium

---

❹

Higher Calorie/Low Cholesterol Model Meal

(From typical Fast Food menu)

Orange juice
Quantity: 6 oz
French toast (hold the butter)
Quantity: 1 order
Maple syrup for above
Quantity: 2 tbsp

Milk, low-fat (skim preferable)
Quantity: 1 cup

Estimated Nutrient Evaluation	
	574 calories
	22% calories as fat
	13% calories as protein
	65% calories as carbohydrate
	135 mg cholesterol
	640 mg sodium

❺
Low Sodium Model Meal

(From typical Hotel/Motel menu)

Fresh fruit cup
Quantity: 1 cup
Toast, whole-wheat (spreads on the side)
Quantity: 2 slices
Margarine for above
Quantity: 1 tsp
Jelly for above
Quantity: 1 tbsp
Yogurt, fruited
Quantity: ½ cup

Estimated
Nutrient
Evaluation

495 calories
16% calories as fat
10% calories as protein
74% calories as carbohydrate
29 mg cholesterol
366 mg sodium

*Note: These models were developed to be slightly lower in calories and other major nutrients than model meals in other chapters because breakfast is often a lower calorie meal than dinner or lunch.

*Nutrition information on selected fast food breakfast choices** (see Abbreviation Key, page 299)

FOOD	Total cals	Fat grams	% Cals as fat	% Cals as carbo-hydrate	% Cals as protein	Sodium	Choles-terol
Breakfast Sandwiches							
Egg Croissan'wich (BK)	304	19	57	27	16	637	243
Egg Croissan'wich with bacon (BK)	355	24	61	23	16	762	249
Egg McMuffin (McD)	290	11	35	39	26	740	226
Sausage Crescent (JB)	584	43	66	19	15	1012	187
Breakfast sandwich (W)	370	19	46	36	18	770	200
Biscuits							
Biscuit with sausage and egg (McD)	520	35	60	25	15	1250	275
Biscuit with bacon, egg, and cheese (McD)	440	26	54	30	16	1230	253
Biscuit (W)	320	17	48	46	6	860	trace
Scrambled Eggs							
Scrambled egg platter with bacon and hash browns (BK)	536	36	60	25	15	975	378
Scrambled egg platter (JB)	662	40	54	31	15	1188	354
Omelette (only)							
Ham, cheese, and mushroom (W)	250	17	61	10	29	405	450
Mushroom, green pepper, and onion (W)	210	15	63	12	25	200	400
Pancakes/French Toast							
(without syrup unless indicated)							
French toast sticks (BK)	499	29	53	39	8	498	74
French toast (W)	400	19	43	46	11	850	115
Pancake platter (JB)	612	22	33	57	10	888	99
Hotcakes with butter and syrup (McD)	410	9	20	72	8	640	21
Syrup—1½ tbsp (JB)	121	–	–	100	–	6	–
Syrup—1½ tbsp (W)	140	–	–	100	–	5	–
Danish							
Great Danish (BK)	500	36	64	32	4	288	6
Apple (McD)	390	18	41	53	6	370	25
Cheese Danish (W)	430	21	44	48	8	500	N/A

Nutrition information on selected fast food breakfast choices (continued)*

FOOD	Total cals	Fat grams	% Cals as fat	% Cals as carbo- hydrate	% Cals as protein	Sodium	Choles- terol
Potatoes							
Hash browns (BK)	162	11	62	32	5	193	2
Hash browns (JB)	116	7	55	38	7	211	3
Breakfast potatoes (W)	360	22	55	41	4	745	20
Juice—6 oz							
Orange juice (W)	80	–	–	95	5	trace	–
Orange juice (BK)	82	–	–	97	3	2	–

Abbreviation Key:

BK	Burger King	McD	McDonald's
JB	Jack-in-the-Box	W	Wendy's

*References used throughout chapter for nutrition evaluation:
1. Specific company information: most currently available information utilized, 1986–present. For more information, see the names, addresses, and phone numbers for each company at the end of Chapter 14, "Healthier Eating Out: Fast Food Style."
2. Composition of Foods: "Fast Foods," United States Department of Agriculture, Human Nutrition Information Service, *Agricultural Handbook 8-21,* 1988.

18

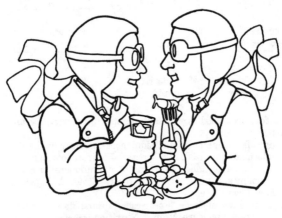

Healthier eating out
Airline Style

The average airline meal is not one to write home about. In fact, the highest expectation for an airline meal is simply something edible, possibly tasty, that will fill you up until you reach your destination. A *Fortune Magazine* article entitled "Why Is Airline Food So Terrible?" describes an airline meal this way: "Lurking beneath that glutinous gravy is meat (origin unknown); gray, ancient-looking peas; a few sad, spindly grains of rice. And don't forget the inevitable hockey-puck hard rolls suitable for use as a blunt instrument." Few air travelers have high hopes for a four-star meal because more times than not they've been disappointed. As the article "Better Airline Fare" in July, 1987, *Health Magazine* exclaimed: "No one ventures 30,000 feet in the air in search of a gastronomic experience."

Certainly airline food has and continues to receive its knocks, and for the most part deservedly so. However, in their defense, providing food service to many people at minimal cost in a crowded plane without the conveniences of most kitchens is quite a difficult task at best. Think about it—the food you consume in the air is prepared on the ground in large food service facilities hours before departure. The hot foods are partially cooked, then cooled and possibly frozen. They are stored until flight time, then reheated on the aircraft prior to being placed on the cart to be delivered to passengers. It's a given that with these constraints, airline meals will never be ones for the record books.

Another criticism of airline food is that, in general, it's not very healthy. From peanuts, the expected handout with your beverage, to creamy salad dressings and thick gravies, airline foods are often laden with fat and salt. A redeeming factor is that the portions are quite small, so even if you eat a high percentage of calories as fat, you're not eating that many calories.

Not long ago one of my clients was attempting to adjust to the hard-to swallow information that to control his weight he simply had to eat much less food. Around that time, he took a trip that included air travel. He returned, stating that he now realized that his portions should be the size of airline meals. "That's a great observation," I stated. "Keep that visual image in mind."

Healthier airline cuisine

Though airline food is neither particularly tasty or healthy, the airlines do get credit for becoming more responsive to the health demands of flyers. With more and more people flying, either for business or pleasure, there are more demands for healthier foods. An article entitled "Pie in the Sky" in *Savvy Magazine*, October, 1988, stated that a survey sponsored by Gallup and several concerned food service groups found that "it was frequent flyers who displayed the greatest unhappiness with airline food .... Almost three-quarters of the passengers surveyed agreed that the airlines should offer more meals with lighter, natural ingredients."

Well, their wish for healthier meals served on airplanes has been granted. In actuality people have been ordering special-diet meals on planes for several years. Low calorie, low cholesterol, low sodium, diabetic, and other special meals have been available for quite a while. More recently, many airlines have tried harder to improve the healthiness of their standard fare—from less salty snack foods to more chicken and fish and less gooey desserts. But they certainly still have a way to go in the taste and health departments.

Probably the best kept secret about airline food is that anyone can order a special meal on most of the major domestic carriers—from vegetarian to low cholesterol and children's plates. No one needs a medical or religious reason for ordering any one of the special meals. And there is no additional charge. All you need is a phone and a voice. Obviously, the airlines are not waving the flag to promote the availability of special meals, though the word is beginning to spread. The article in the October, 1988, issue of *Savvy Magazine* stated that "about 3 percent of all airline meals are special orders, and the trend is growing . . . ."

Special meals are available

There's an amazing array of special meals available. Some of the special-diet offerings are diabetic, low calorie (though they don't state the number of calories), low cholesterol, low sodium, and bland. For people who avoid certain foods due to personal preference or for religious reasons, there are vegetarian meals, kosher, and several airlines even provide Hindu, Oriental, and Muslim meals. For the young traveler, infants', toddlers', and children's meals are available from certain airlines when ordered in advance.

Possibly the best choice on airlines (as I'm quickly discovering) is the fruit or seafood plate. These are often better choices because they're served cold. There is less taste and palatibility damage done to cold food than hot when it's held for a long time. Even if you're on a low cholesterol, fat, or sodium meal plan, the fruit or seafood might be a better choice than the special meal. It most likely will fit into your guidelines and taste better as well.

The fruit plate can range from simply an array of fresh fruit to fruit with cottage cheese and/or yogurt and crackers. The seafood plate might be shrimp or seafood salad, served with greens, dressing, and crackers. These are very nice light alternatives to the overcooked vegetables and thick, brown gravies. Watch out though—you'll have the other passengers staring at your tray with desiring eyes. They might angrily ask how you managed to get that. Be nice and take a minute to give them some healthy advice.

Several airlines claim to be working in consultation with dietitians to improve their menus. According to a phone contact at American Airlines, they have developed heart-healthy meals called the American Traveler Menu in consultation with the Cooper (Ken Cooper, M.D.) Clinic in Dallas. There are six meal choices available for breakfast, lunch, or dinner (if a meal is being served on the flight); these change monthly and are in line with the nutrition recommendations of the American Heart Association. According to the October, 1988, issue of *Savvy Magazine,* Northwest Airlines is working with nutritionists to revise and improve their special meals. So, obviously, the airlines are listening, and healthier foods in the air are simply a phone call away.

The "how-to" of ordering special meals

It's surprisingly simple to have a special meal waiting with your name on it as your plane taxis down the runway. Most of the airlines specify that you provide at least 24-hours notice for special meals. It's easiest to order the special meals when you make reservations. For frequent flyers who consistently use the same travel agent, just specify which meal you want when you make your call. They will list it in your record as they do the non-smoking section and seat preferences.

It's important to realize that if you've ordered a special meal, you might have to wait until the end of food service to receive it, or maybe you'll be lucky and get served first. Sometimes you need to make the steward or stewardess aware that you have ordered a special meal. They might request that you identify yourself at the beginning of the food service.

Also be ready to have your special order fouled up. Personally, I've had no problem so far, but you should be on the ready for the unexpected. As with any special request, you increase the chance of having one of the many steps it takes to get the meal go wrong. You might want to make an extra call to make sure that your special request has been entered into the computer system.

Beverages and snacks

Most flyers know that they will at least be served a beverage. The free choices are generally consistent from airline to airline—coffee, tea, carbonated beverages, mineral waters, and juices. If you are choosing a hot beverage and want to add cream, be careful of the definition of cream. They might have the non-dairy powders or liquid whiteners that often contain coconut oil. A bit of whole or low-fat (preferable) milk is a better and often an available choice. Alternative sweeteners are always on board. The usual is a saccharin-based sweetener, but more airlines are making Equal®, the NutraSweet®-brand sweetener available. If your preference is Equal, you'd better take it along with you on your travels because it's not always available.

As for cold beverages, if you're carefully monitoring calories, you're best off with the low-calorie carbonated ones, club soda, or mineral waters—all of which usually are in large supply. Tomato juice or my favorite, Bloody Mary mix (hold the vodka), are also low-calorie choices. Juices are alternatives, but don't forget a 12-ounce can of juice can run up to almost 200 calories. Read through Chapter 19 on choosing beverages for more information on alcoholic and non-alcoholic beverages.

On many flights a small bag of peanuts, salted or honey-coated, will be placed on your tray with your beverage. These delicious little nuggets are a bit of protein loaded with fat. You're better off purchasing a small bag of pretzels or popcorn prior to boarding the plane, or just say "no thanks" to the bag of peanuts.

On flights of one to two hours but not within particular meal times, you might be served a snack. Sometimes the snacks are more palatable than the hot meal. Again, it's likely due to the fact that these foods are not cooked, frozen, and then reheated prior to serving. Snacks usually include a small sandwich with meat and cheese or crackers and cheese. Fruit, chocolates, or cookies are also often included. Some airlines do have special diet snacks. To find out, simply ask when you're making reservations.

Take charge of your in-flight nutrition

The first rule of thumb in air travel is to expect the unexpected. The second is to have a sense of humor and "go with the flow." The third rule is synonymous with the Boy Scout motto, "Always Be Prepared."

To establish that sense of control when traveling through the skies, don't leave it up to the airlines as to what and when you'll be served. Before you board the plane, in fact several hours before, think about your travel eating plan. This is crucially important for people who have diabetes and are on insulin or oral medications to control blood sugar. It is critically important for people who have diabetes not to leave things to chance. The rule of being prepared for anything must be followed.

If you will need or want something to eat in flight, you might wish to purchase something prior to arriving at the airport, or buy it at the airport, although you will pay more. There is absolutely no problem taking food onto the plane. I've done it plenty of times, and no one has said a word. Of course, you can't eat during takeoff or landing.

Here are a few portable suggestions for healthier snacks: bag of pretzels, soft pretzel (often sold in airports), bag of popcorn or fresh-popped popcorn, fresh fruit, low-fat yogurt, and low-fat crackers. If you will be on a long flight or simply are ready to eat more than the plane will have to offer, try bringing a sandwich along or purchasing one at the airport. If it's breakfast time, either a portable muffin or bagel should do the trick.

Standard airline fare probably will not improve dramatically in the near future. Maybe there'll be small changes due to the demand for healthier food choices. The best policy is to take control. Go the healthy route, take advantage of the special meals, and order ahead. If you don't want to partake of airline fare at all, preplan and make your purchases prior to boarding.

19

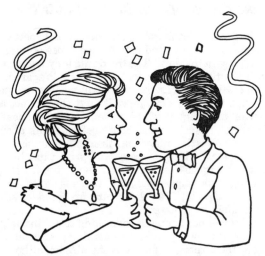

Choosing beverages
Alcoholic and Non-Alcoholic

I n many dining situations the first question you are asked is, "May I bring you something to drink?" In some restaurants the choices may simply be a soda, glass of milk, coffee, or water. However, in many dining spots the choice of beer or wine is added, and in yet others the whole gamut of beverages from water to distilled spirits to brandy or liqueur is offered before, during, and after the meal. Since beverages are an integral part of eating out and because lots of calories and unhealthy dietary components can be contributed by beverages, you need to be prepared with a plan and a response to the question, "May I bring you something to drink?"

Whether you decide on an alcoholic beverage, sweetened soda (or "pop" as it's called in many locales), fruit juice, or mineral water, there are several factors to consider, both medical and nutritional. For instance, is alcohol appropriate in view of your particular medical condition, such as an elevated blood triglyceride level, is a large fruit juice a good choice for someone with diabetes, or is a regular soda or two beers a sensible selection if you are trying to lose a few pounds.

Because all beverages are simply liquids, there is a tendency to forget you are consuming calories. Unfortunately, that's far from true; there are a lot of calories in many beverages—alcoholic or not. You'll find that a regular soda (12 oz) contains about 140 calories and offers nothing but sugar; a regular beer also contains about 140 calories and offers little in the way of nutrition. An 8-oz glass of orange juice adds 110 calories but does, of course, provide some vitamins and minerals. Due to the potentially large number of calories and other unhealthy ingredients that may be found in drinks, beverage selections need to be made carefully, keeping health and nutrition factors in mind.

ALCOHOLIC BEVERAGES

Medical and health considerations

There certainly are medical and health factors to consider when making the decision to select an alcoholic beverage. Over the last several years, there has been much publicity surrounding drinking and driving, and most people are aware of the connection between heavy alcohol consumption and liver disease. People are less aware of the relationship between heavy alcohol consumption and cancer of the mouth, esophagus, liver, and colon, which was discussed in the Diet and Health Summary conducted under auspices of the National Research Council and published in 1989. This research group also drew a correlation between excessive alcohol intake and an increased occurence of heart disease, high blood pressure, stroke, and osteoporosis. Obviously, alcohol has its negative effects on health.

From a general good health and nutrition perspective, moderation is the magic word when it comes to alcohol consumption. As stated, heavy imbibing is correlated with many diseases. It is also well known that you'd be hard pressed to find much nutritional value in alcohol. In fact, excessive alcohol intake, in lieu of adequate food consumption, is known to result in nutrient deficiencies.

The positive, healthy aspects of moderate alcohol consumption have been connected with stress reduction and modestly raising HDLs—the "good" cholesterol (high density lipoproteins). However, with all aspects considered, most health professionals would not make the recommendation to start drinking or to increase alcohol consumption just to derive those benefits. That holds true especially in light of the minimal nutritional benefits and excess calories found in alcoholic drinks.

People attempting to lose weight or maintain their newly found waistlines should practice strict moderation when it comes to alcohol, if not abstinence on most occasions. You simply can't afford the calories. If you are trying to keep calories in the range of 1,200 per day and you choose to have 100–200 calories worth of alcohol several times a week, you certainly will have to curtail somewhere and probably wind up sacrificing the nutrients obtained from highly nutritious foods.

Beer

It might be labeled Singha in Thai restaurants, Tsing Tsao in Chinese restaurants, Dos Equis in Mexican eating spots, and Bud or Mich when eating American style. But basically beer is beer, whether it is from Thailand or brewed here in the U.S. Beer is a brewed and fermented drink. Its taste is created from blending malted barley and other starches and flavoring the brew with hops. Interestingly, *sake*, a Japanese drink, is a refermented brewed beverage made from rice.

There are very few differences nutritionally and calorically from one beer to the next. Bottom line—the calories add up fast. A 12-oz can of regular beer contains about 150 calories. And how many people drink just one? With beer, there certainly is an alternative: light beer. Most light beers ring in at about 100 calories for 12 oz. Obviously, that can add up quickly, too, but it might be a helpful alternative when trying to minimize calories.

Wine

Whether it's red, white, or rosé, domestic, French, or Italian, wine contains about 120 calories for 6 oz. So, if you really like red wine better than white or fruity wine better than dry, the best advice is to drink less but drink what you enjoy. Light wine has been made available in supermarkets, but it does not seem to appear on menus in restaurants. If you are used to splitting a bottle of wine, you might want to reduce the quantity you consume by simply ordering a half-carafe or ordering by the glass. Today, many restaurants offer a selection of better wines by the glass rather than simply the house red or white, which are often unexciting.

A few suggestions about wine. Always make sure you have a non-caloric beverage by your side along with the glass of wine. That way, you can use the non-caloric beverage to quench your thirst and you are more likely to sip the wine, making it last longer. If you wish to limit yourself to one glass of wine and you really enjoy it with your meal, don't order it until the meal arrives. Order a non-caloric beverage to accompany your dining companions as they sip their alcoholic drinks.

Another calorie-conscious strategy is to order a wine spritzer, again white, red, or rosé doesn't matter. A wine spritzer is made with wine, club soda, and a twist or lemon or lime. I'll often order a spritzer and request that the bartender mix it half and half rather than the usual three-fourths wine and one-fourth soda. What's nice about a spritzer is that you get a nice, tall, thirst-quenching drink with a small amount of wine and thus limited calories. So, for the same number of calories in one glass of wine, you can have two wine spritzers.

Try to avoid spritzers made with sweetened soda, wine punches with juices, or wine coolers; the "mixes" in all of these add calories. It is common to find sangria by the pitcher in Mexican restaurants. Sangria is best avoided due to the extra calories from additional ingredients such as fruit juices and granulated sugar. These items should definitely be avoided by those with diabetes due to their high sugar content.

Champagne is actually classified as wine. Champagne, which is named after its origins in Cham-

pagne, France, is most often used as a celebratory
beverage. It's used to toast an occasion. Small quantities are usually consumed. Champagne is slightly
higher in calories than most wines, and the calories
are somewhat dependent on how dry it is. Drier champagne is slightly higher in calories. Another place
champagne is often seen is at brunches, or in
mimosas, where it is teamed with orange juice.

Distilled spirits

Rum, gin, vodka, and whiskey are all classified as
distilled spirits. Interestingly, like wine, they all have
the same number of calories—about 100 per jigger (1½
oz) for 80-proof liquor. Many people have the misconception that rum, scotch, and bourbon are higher in
calories than gin and vodka. That misconception
might relate to the fact that these distilled spirits are
often found in sweeter drinks or taste slightly sweeter
and more concentrated than vodka and gin. Actually,
100 calories per shot is not bad when compared to the
calories of other alcoholic beverages. So if hard liquor
is what you prefer, don't get caught up in the misconception that wine and beer have less calories. But certainly you get more volume for your calories with
wine and beer.

The bigger problem with distilled spirits is that they
are often mixed with other high-calorie ingredients.
Consider a tequila sunrise made with tequila, orange
juice, and grenadine (a sweet, red syrup), or a rusty
nail made with Drambuie and scotch. These drinks
are closer to the 150–200 calorie range. It's best to
avoid drinks that are a combination of distilled spirits
and another liquor, cordial, fruit juices, sugar, sweetened soda, tonic water, or cream. Think about ordering a vodka, rum, gin, or whiskey on the rocks, with
a splash of water, club soda, or diet soda. Diet tonic
water is also produced but not often stocked in most
restaurant bars.

Liqueur and brandy

The last category of alcoholic beverages is liqueurs,
cordials, and brandies. Liqueurs and cordials synony-
mously describe beverages such as the familiar Kahlua, Amaretto, and Drambuie. These drinks are most
commonly used straight as an after-dinner drink or
in combination with other distilled spirits in a mixed

drink. Brandy is created from distilled wine or the mash of fruit. The most familiar brandy is cognac, but other popular examples are Greek Metaxa and kirsch (a cherry brandy).

Liqueurs, cordials, and brandies ring in at about 150 calories per jigger (1½ oz), a substantial number of calories for a small quantity. They are often consumed in addition to other alcoholic beverages, following a meal. However, if you decide that is what you want and you have "budgeted" the calories, then sip away slowly.

Another way to enjoy these beverages and get more volume for your calories is to use a liqueur as part of a coffee drink, such as Irish coffee or café royale. By adding black coffee to a shot of liqueur, you increase the volume substantially. Ask the waitperson to hold the whipped cream and sugar, which are often added to these after-dinner coffee drinks. If you can use one of these after-dinner concoctions to quench your sweet tooth, that's great. As others are downing their mega-calorie confections, you are sipping a 150-calorie, no-fat, no-cholesterol dessert.

NON-ALCOHOLIC BEVERAGES

From our review of alcoholic beverages, it is clear that calories from any type of alcohol add up quickly, and it is often difficult to limit the quantity consumed, for a variety of reasons. In some dining-out situations it might make more sense to eliminate the alcohol and enjoy a hot or cold non-alcoholic beverage. If you choose to consume alcohol, it is still wise to intermingle one or two non-caloric hot or cold beverages to help quench your thirst. For instance, have a club soda with your meal and coffee or tea afterward.

Another positive side to drinking non-caloric beverages is that they help fill you up. This is an especially helpful strategy for weight watchers who are trying to minimize food intake. If you work on forcing yourself to put down the knife and fork and sip a beverage, you'll fill up faster and in the end consume fewer calories.

Cold beverages

The most common cold beverages are the variety of sodas, or pop. Regular sweetened and low-calorie sodas are listed on most menus. There is often a mix of juices such as orange, apple, grapefruit, or tomato. Iced tea and coffee are frequently available, and milk is commonly found in the beverage column.

The type of milk is often undefined on the menu. It is up to you to ask about the type of milk on hand. Many times only whole milk is available, but more restaurants today are responding to consumer demand and stock either 2 percent or skim milk. Actually, it is important that you continue to ask for the lower-fat milk because, hopefully, the more it is requested, the quicker the manager will put it on the menu. In fact, some fast food restaurants have responded to the need and already have added lower-fat milk to menu offerings.

If the restaurant has a bar, it is more likely you will be able to order non-caloric mineral water, such as Perrier, Evian, or club soda. You might flavor these with a twist or piece of lemon or lime. Don't forget about good old water. It is obviously non-caloric. One idea to make water a bit more enticing is to request a piece of lemon or lime to squeeze into your water glass. If you like lemonade, you can easily make your own at your table by using a few drops of fresh lemon and a sugar substitute to sweeten it up.

Iced tea and iced coffee make great refreshing beverages that initially are non-caloric. Be careful that you don't add enough milk, cream, or sugar to push up the calories. Fresh-brewed iced tea is great plain or with a few drops of lemon; sweeten it up with a sugar substitute.

Sugar-sweetened sodas, the most frequently ordered beverage by the American public, should definitely be avoided. As you can see from the nutrient information table that follows, a 12-oz glass of soda provides about 140 calories. That's a chunk, especially when you realize that you are simply consuming sugar and water. There is basically no nutritional value in the 140 calories. That would represent 10 percent of the calories allowed on a 1,400-calorie meal plan. Spending 10 percent on one can of sugar water would not be my choice. I'd rather have a large baked potato or a bigger portion of my entree, something that provides volume and nutrition.

Fruit juice is certainly a healthy alternative. Orange, apple, or grapefruit are all nutrient-dense choices. However, they also represent high-calorie alternatives when you consider that you are simply quenching your thirst and helping your food go down. A mere 6 oz of juice holds about 80 calories, with apple being a bit higher. My choice would be to eat a piece of fruit to get some food volume and fiber. Consider having a half-grapefruit or sliced banana on cereal for breakfast rather than automatically ordering juice.

Hot beverages

The most commonly listed hot beverages, served from breakfast to midnight snack time are coffee and tea. Many restaurants offer brewed decaffeinated coffee and more are beginning to offer decaffeinated tea. When choosing coffee or tea, whether regular or decaffeinated, you start off with essentially zero calories; but the calories can creep up when scoops of sugar and cream are added. Be careful that you are minimizing sugar or using a sugar substitute, and use milk rather than cream in your coffee, especially if you like light coffee.

More interesting teas are being served in many restaurants today, not simply the standard blends. In better restaurants it's common to find my favorites, Earl Grey, English Breakfast, or Darjeeling tea. More often of late, a variety of herbal teas are listed on menus: lemon, orange and spice, and red zinger are just a few. The great thing about herbal teas is that they are caffeine-free and have a lovely mellow flavor.

A hot beverage that is usually available at fancier restaurants is espresso. Espresso has its roots in Italy and typically follows the meal there. It has been integrated into better dining establishments in America. Some would define espresso as power-packed coffee. Espresso is very, very rich coffee, which is enjoyable after a meal. It is most often served in a demitasse that at most holds 3–4 ozs. A twist of lemon is run over the brim of the cup, and sugar cubes often accompany espresso. Both the lemon and sugar cut the bitter taste. It's a nice way to end a meal and maybe something different if you have never tried it. Best yet, there are minimal calories, no fat, and no cholesterol!

Eating out has become a major activity in today's fast-paced world. Hopefully, this book will provide you with the knowledge and skill to make it a healthful as well as a pleasurable experience.

For further information

American Diabetes Association
National Service Center
1660 Duke Street
Alexandria, VA 22314
800-ADA-DISC

American Dietetic Association
Nutrition Resources
216 W. Jackson Boulevard, Suite 800
Chicago, IL 60606
312-899-0040, ext. 4853

American Heart Association
National Center
7320 Greenville Avenue
Dallas, TX 75231
800-527-6941

National Heart, Lung, and Blood
Institute Information Center
4733 Bethesda Avenue, Suite 530
Bethesda, MD 20814

The NHLBI has several programs that provide information and educational materials: NHLBI Smoking Education Program Information Center; National Cholesterol Education Program; National High Blood Pressure Education Program.